The Joy of
Weight Loss

A Spiritual Guide to Easy Fitness

Norris J. Chumley

Foreword by Harville Hendrix, Ph.D. and Helen LaKelly Hunt, MA, MLA
Preface by Monica Sweeney, MD, MPH
Illustrations by Catherine Stine

My love is my weight.
—*Saint Augustine*

LANTERN BOOKS
A Division of Booklight Inc.

2001
Lantern Books
One Union Square West, Suite 201
New York, NY 10003

No single approach to weight loss works for everyone. I urge you to consult with your physician before making any significant changes in your eating habits or physical activities to ensure that what you propose for yourself is nutritionally sound, safe, and healthy.

This book contains food and activity plans that are not intended for pregnant or nursing women, or if you have any health problems or diseases.

Printed in the United States of America

Library of Congress Cataloging-in-Publication Data

Chumley, Norris J.
    The joy of weight loss : a spiritual guide to easy fitness / Norris J. Chumley ; foreword by Harville Hendrix and Helen LaKelly Hunt; preface by Monica Sweeney; illustrations by Catherine Stine.
    p. cm.
    ISBN 1-930051-19-0 (alk. paper)
    1. Weight loss. 2. Weight loss—Psychological aspects. I. Title

RM222.2 C485 2001
613.7—dc21

00-066320

Book design by Richard Oriolo
Jacket design by Jack Ribik
Photographs by Robert Baldridge

First and foremost, this book is for God.

Thank you for my life, the many rescues and blessings, and the Joy of Weight Loss.

Dedicated to my wife Catherine, and our children Jack and Nate.

To my family: Gary, Hays, A., and Ross Chumley, Edna Chumley Henderson, Dorothy Stine, Richard and Lou Stine, John and Karen Stine, and all of my other aunts, uncles, nieces and nephews, cousins and in-laws. God bless you and thank you all.

In memory of Georgia Deal, and in honor of the Deal family.

In memory of my parents Mary Ellen Chumley and Norris Gary Chumley.

Special Thanks ⤳

Those who made this book real:
Gene Gollogly
Martin Rowe
Carole Sinclair
Michael Fragnito
Daniel L. Rabinowitz
Monica Sweeney, MD, MPH
Juliet H. Campbell, MS, CDN, CNS

Lifelong True Friends:
Scott Alber and Barbara Hatton Alber
Donn and Ruth Alber
Robert Eckert
Carol Nordberg
Matt and Nancy Ferro Baker
Frank Haney
Neil Sharrow
Michael White
Bob and Mary Kline
Harville Hendrix
Helen LaKelly Hunt

Those who believe in me:
Jesus, Moses, Muhammad, Krishna
    and Buddha
Shrii Shrii Anandamurtiji
T George Harris
Stephen Mitchell
Al Cattabiani
Curtis and Julie Davis
Bob and Marjorie Davis
Paul and Glenna Pack
Mary Sarkes and Tom Tarzian
Dan Yankelovitch and Barbara Lee
Norman Lear
David Mallery
Jan Miller
Benjamin Robin
Suzanne Bevier
Fred A. Billings
Abby Saxon
Alan Eisner
Jamahl and Amity Black
Alex Hood
Howard Siegel, MD

Susan Sarandon

Deepak Chopra

Arielle Ford

Thomas Moore

Ram Dass

Abby Saxon

Marina Goldshteyn

Janice Kamrin

Dan Crystal

Jared Blaut

Greg Wigfall

Gail Stentiford

Dan Cordle

Scott Willet

New York University Coles
Recreation Center

New York Quarterly Meeting of the
Religious Society of Friends

Don Kautz

Arlene Feinblatt

Joan Avalone

Donna in the coffee shop

Kelly at the Library

My friends from the men's group

Bedford-Stuyvesant Family
Health Center

The Joy of Weight Loss Groups

The cab driver who heard my story and
told me to write it down

Contents

Preface xi

Foreword xv

One: How I Found The Joy of Weight Loss 1

Two: Finding and Allowing Joy 16

Three The Joy of Weight Loss Personal Program 24

    Part I: The Joy of Surrender 24

    Part II: Eat Healthily And Be Active 38

    Part III: Joy Assured 76

Four: Joy, Continued 87

Five: The Joy of Weight Loss Daily Companion 96

Appendix A: The Joy of Weight Loss Menu Ideas 171

Appendix B: The Joy of Weight Loss Daily Checklist 179

Citations 181

by Monica Sweeney, MD

Dr. Monica Sweeney has lost two dress sizes and stayed a reasonable weight for over fifteen years on her own variation of "The Joy of Weight Loss." She is Vice President and Medical Director, Bedford-Stuyvesant Family Health Center, Brooklyn, NY, past President, Kings County Medical Society, and a member of the Public Health Committee of the New York State Medical Society.

When one thinks of illnesses and diseases that result from obesity, most people think of heart disease, high blood pressure, and diabetes. We refer to these as the big three. But the list is very long and includes: depression/social isolation, arthritis/back pain, pulmonary embolus (blood clots from the legs, thighs, to the lungs), gallbladder disease, sleep apnea, infertility in women, increased cancer risk in men and women, chronic lack of energy, etc. For over twenty years I have practiced medicine in New York City. From the beginning, my focus has been on disease prevention and health promotion through healthier life styles. These strategies have included stopping smoking, exercising regularly, and losing weight.

I'm really sorry I didn't have a complete guide to weight loss like Norris Chumley's *The Joy of Weight Loss* when I began my program. Long before obesity was reclassified by the American Heart Association as a major modifiable risk factor to prevent heart disease, I would tell my patients: "I can't help you unless you help yourself; this is a partnership."

The story of just one of my patients stands out, because he only needed the message once. The patient, who is a judge who had been recommended to me by a surgeon friend of mine, complained of severe shortness of breath, especially when walking, chest pain, and indigestion—just to mention a few problems. After I had obtained a complete history and conducted a physical examination, making sure he didn't already have heart disease, I began to give him his exit consultation. He interrupted and said: "Other than the fact I'm overweight, what else is 'wrong with me'?"

"Nothing else," I said. I explained that his blood pressure was high and that his sugar was high, but that the best treatment for all his symptoms was to lose 100 pounds. I then told him that if he didn't lose weight, he should select the suit in which he wished to be buried. He left the office without making the recommended follow-up appointment. A few years later at a social gathering held by the same surgeon friend I was introduced to a handsome young man who said to me: "You should remember people whose life you saved." It was the judge. He had lost the 100 pounds and, with the loss, all his medical problems had gone.

I have hundreds of success stories about people who changed their lives by losing twenty pounds or so. The latest medical evidence confirms great health improvements with modest weight loss. If I had had a tool like *The Joy of Weight Loss*, maybe some of my failures would have been successes. But I'm thankful that it's available now to millions of overweight Americans. Restrictive dieting is not the answer. Losing weight is easy; keeping it off is the hard part. The best "diet" to accomplish this goal is a varied and well-balanced diet, eaten in moderation for life. That's the plan in *The Joy of Weight Loss*.

In addition to food self-management, exercising regularly is the other essential part of the program. I tell my patients: find an enjoyable activity, schedule it into your daily routine, and stay with it. I walk around Prospect Park with a friend early in the morning for about an hour. That hour is one of my greatest daily pleasures. When I can't walk because I have an early train or plane, I feel very deprived. My energy level decreases, my sleep and elimination are impaired, and in the end I just have to go for a walk.

I myself have used *The Joy of Weight Loss* weight loss program. Food used to control me. When I was sad I would eat; when I was tired I would eat; when I was celebrating I would eat; when I was angry I would eat. I was unwilling to accept that anymore; so I made the decision that I wasn't going to let it happen and…something snapped. "Enough of this already," I said. I did then what is a fundamental component of *The Joy of Weight Loss*'s success as a program. I sought God's help.

I had a real burden and so I got rid of the burden. I didn't do it by myself. I became more spiritual, thinking more about seeing myself in a different place. I thought about my father a lot during this period and how he used to talk about overcoming obstacles. He wasn't talking about weight, but he was talking about faith and having faith to solve problems. His faith was in the scriptural passage: "Faith is the substance of things hoped for, the evidence of things not seen." I decided I could lose weight based on that message; I just had to have faith that I could do it with God's help.

That really was the turning point. It had to do with turning my will over to a higher power.

Developing good habits is the second key step after surrendering your will to a higher power. During my journey, once the idea of putting my faith to work for my weight problem came into my consciousness, it was easy to surrender my will—it's what I had done so many times for other things. Believe me, surrendering is easy after many, many failures. I have always incorporated my patients' spiritual beliefs into their medical care. Once you surrender your will to a higher power, you will immediately feel better.

I have been on a version of *The Joy of Weight Loss* program for years. It works! I eat all the foods I like in smaller amounts. Over the years, I've learned how to let go of unhealthy habits that would jeopardize my achieving health and happiness. I don't weigh myself (I haven't for years); but I wear the same size clothing since I lost two dress sizes years ago. I exercise by walking four miles four to five times a week. The most important part of my journey is that I no longer eat to feel joy. My life is full of joy though my faith in God.

I call it a burden shared, but you can call it what you will. At heart, *The Joy of Weight Loss* is a two-step program: Surrender to your higher power and feel the joy while losing weight.

I try and become centered, to see God in me and in everyone. That helps me also with other problems, because I don't take out my frustration on food now. If you listen to that little voice inside, you'll be guided rightly—something that's true with so many things and food. Now I know how much to eat; I eat more sensibly, and for the right reasons. I have proof: God helped me!

by Harville Hendrix, Ph.D. and Helen LaKelly Hunt, M.A., M. L. A.

Dr. Harville Hendrix and his partner and wife, Helen LaKelly Hunt, have written many books on relationships, including the bestselling Getting The Love You Want, A Guide for Couples. *Their pioneering work combines pastoral psychotherapy, spirituality, life experience, and the practice of empathy in a profoundly effective approach to wholeness called Imago Relationship Therapy. A television and media-workshop series, "Getting The Love You Want," based on their work was produced and co-written by Norris Chumley, and introduced by Oprah Winfrey.*

⬿ When we were asked to write a foreword to this book, we were initially puzzled, because we are not experts in the field. Our area of expertise is relationships, specifically the relationship between committed partners and between parents and children. At first, we could not see how we could comment on a book outside our field of competence. On second thought, however, it occurred to us that everyone has a relationship to food, and that relationship includes some of the same unconscious dynamics that influence our selection of an intimate partner. We have learned, for instance, that our selection of a partner is influenced by our relationship with our parents, although we do not consciously know that. When we meet someone who is similar in significant ways to our parents, we unconsciously select them as a love partner. It is called falling in love, and has addictive qualities, like our love of food. We engage in a power struggle with our partner to establish our identity and role and, if we are lucky, we finally become conscious and co-create a loving and durable relationship. If we do not become conscious, we continue in the struggle for a lifetime or change partners.

Our relationship to food follows the same sequence. We tend to love the foods we had in childhood, but often do not know that. Food takes on a symbolic meaning and we engage in eating rituals. We wonder how anyone could love other kinds of foods, especially our partner. We struggle with food, sometimes feeling it is in charge of us. Or we try to change our relationship to food, often succeeding, but most often failing. If we become conscious of our food identity and our food addiction, we learn how and what to eat for our best welfare. If we do not, food becomes our friend when we are down or our enemy when we are overweight. Unlike our intimate partner, whom we may choose to keep or divorce, we have a life-long relationship to food. Becoming conscious of our food addiction is as important as becoming conscious in personal relationships.

Our second concern is that we do not have a weight problem, although Harville has been concerned a bit about his middle age spread, and Helen had some weight concerns in her early years. Because of that, occasionally we look at diet books to see what new ways are being devised to lose weight. Essentially, our observation is that most of them are distinguished by whether they focus on protein or carbohydrates. These two issues are surrounded by what can be called esoteric suggestions such as starting the day with fruit, eliminating refined sugar, and how to alternate eating certain foods to aid digestion. Some diet programs have philosophies about how we should follow evolutionary eating habits while others take a biological and chemical approach to the body; some take a psychological approach to the meaning of food and its function in our lives while others relate weight-gain to stress and life style. What is common to them all is that any diet must be accompanied by various amounts of exercise, calorie reduction, drinking eight glasses of water daily, and stress reduction. What is interesting about this is omitting these four items renders any diet ineffective.

From an analytical point of view, most diet books tend to treat weight gain as a symptom and tend not to deal with causes. Therefore, the message is to eliminate the symptom of weight gain by engaging in a weight loss program. This book is the first one we have seen that offers a different perspective. Norris Chumley is a veteran of weight loss. As you will learn from his personal sharing in the following pages, he has lost a significant amount of weight and kept it off. He has learned a secret that he boldly shares with the reader. From his perspective, weight gain is a spiritual problem. For him, food becomes a substitute for one's relationship to God. Over-eating is an attempt to fill the void created by unfulfilled and unconscious spiritual yearning. Chumley's research indicates that the chronic pattern of gaining and losing weight, which happens with all diet plans, can be overcome only when one comes to terms with the Divine Reality that enfolds us all. When our relationship to God is resolved, our relationship with food will be transformed and the problem of weight will disappear as a concern. And we will be the weight we are supposed to be.

While weight has not been a major symptom in our lives, there are other ways in which we have, at times, slipped out of balance. We now see this, as Chumley does, as a wake up call for realignment. The same is true for couples with whom we work. We have also learned what the author has identified: that most of our significant struggles, with food or with our partner, constitute a spiritual process. To become rightly aligned with our partner and with food requires us to reconnect with the Divine Source.

This is a truly remarkable and revolutionary point of view for a diet book, and anyone who has struggled with weight loss will find this a rewarding and fulfilling path. The symptom will disappear when the cause is addressed.

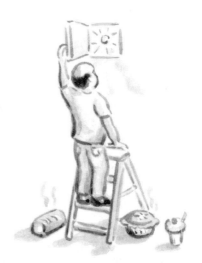

One

How I Found
The Joy of Weight Loss

For twenty-two years all I wanted to do was eat. I couldn't stop thinking about the next snack or the next meal.

Food was my only comfort to help fill the emptiness I felt inside. Today, right now, at this moment, I'm 160 pounds lighter than I used to be. It's been over eleven years since I had a weight problem. I have finally succeeded in losing weight and keeping it off. I have found real happiness and joy in my life. I can handle any problem that comes my way and I don't just depend on food for comfort and fulfillment anymore. I am one of God's true living miracles, and this is my story. I offer it to you because I know that you, too, can be one of God's living miracles. You too, can rise above your problems and be liberated. And I promise—it'll be a completely joyous experience.

My name is Norris Chumley, but my nickname at school was E. Normous Chubby. I was always overweight. I was born overweight: over thirteen pounds. I was a chubby kid, then I quickly grew to be a fat kid. At age sixteen, I weighed 400 pounds. There wasn't a day that went by that I didn't feel bad about being a fat kid. Because I was so obese, I also felt stupid, invalid, weird, and ugly.

One time, when I was going to take swimming classes, I couldn't stand to be seen in a bathing suit—and I was only five years old! I remember the coach joking about how fat I was and the other kids also laughing at me. It was incredibly painful, week after week, to endure their torture and my own self-hatred. Consequently, I didn't learn to swim until I was thirty-two.

It wasn't as if my family wasn't aware of the problems associated with weight. There wasn't a time that my family wasn't on a crash diet. Every meal would be dry, broiled meat with very little flavor, with tasteless, steamed vegetables. We never had any butter and rarely used any margarine. While we would never have desserts in front of the rest of the family, my mom and I would secretly binge all day and every night. There was constant pressure for us to be thin and perfect, but we never were. We knew we were miserable fat failures. I am telling you about my difficult childhood because I learned to find joy out of misery. If I hadn't had a hard time as a kid, I might never have learned the deep value of joy as an adult. If I hadn't had a severe weight problem, I may never have worked very hard to recover from it. You can use your pain and misery to motivate yourself to change, too. Therefore, I hope you'll share your difficulties with yourself and others. It'll help a lot to open up and get honest about your life.

Eating Together in Secret

My mother was "morbidly obese" (that's the term doctors use for us fat folks) and was probably over 400 pounds herself, although she would never have admitted it. I loved her more than anyone, even more than the food she fed me. She took an extra-special liking to me, I think, because she was so fat and I was a fat little reflection of her. We would eat together in secret. She had chocolate candies hidden in every drawer of the house. There were cookies in places you would never expect, such as in the library, and we had a whole, separate deep freeze full of ice cream. There must have been a hundred pints of ice cream in that deep freeze and we would eat them every day.

In addition to the ice cream I ate during the day, I always ate a pint, sometimes a half-gallon of ice cream *every night* before going to bed. Recently, I looked at the calorie count for just a pint of ice cream and discovered it to be anywhere from 900 to 1500 calories per pint. That's two-thirds the amount of calories a thin person eats in a day.

In addition to food's central role in our family, there was a lot of stress, confrontation, and arguing going on. When he was around, my father would criticize me. I think he was jealous of me. At the dinner table we would complain about how awful things were and what difficult problems we had. It seemed there was rarely anything good ever happening, and if there was it was never good enough. Dad would whip or slap the living daylights out of me for the slightest infraction. I believe he had an addiction problem like my mom and I, except the substance was alcohol. Almost every night I'd have to hold back the tears during supper. Mom knew what was going on, but she couldn't stop it. So she would soothe me (and herself) with another helping.

Dessert: My Mother's Favorite Thing In Life

As you can see, we never really had much fun, and the only comfort in our house was food. About the only fun thing we did together was eat and, since we were always dieting, meals were no joy. I remember my mother saying that she didn't care about drinking, sports, movies, or much of anything else other than dessert. Desserts were her favorite things in life.

To her, there was nothing better than a delicious chocolate cake or an ice cream sundae. My mother and father were constantly telling me I was too fat and that I had to lose weight. My mom had gone on a crash diet when she was in her twenties and had gotten to where she was fairly thin. But then she gained all the weight back. She lamented for years how she could never lose the weight again. Therefore, she was always on a diet.

My mother once dragged me to a commercial weight club when I was twelve. I was not just the only child there, I was the only male. Every eye was on me when I was made to get on the scale week after week. The leaders of the club program had a policy of screaming out loud when someone had lost anything, and the whole room would cheer loudly. I never lost more than one pound in a week, and frequently gained. The silence when I got on the scales was deafening. I wanted to murder those people. I hated them making my mother and me weigh and measure everything, and buy those repulsive and tasteless frozen diet dinners. The whole thing ended in yet another dieting failure after several months of utter torture. The only change was that we were much worse off emotionally than when we began.

It Was Hard to Make Friends

When you're as fat as I was, people don't like to be seen with you, so I didn't have many friends. I was certainly never able to hang out with the kids that were cool. It was hard to make friends and it was very hard to keep friends. A technique I used was to appear very happy, be the class clown, and to be the best listener anyone could ever meet. I would show off my obesity by selling peeks at my giant breasts for a quarter and make fun of myself in order to get laughs and sympathy. But laughs and sympathy were as far as it went, because most kids ultimately treated me like a loser.

The few friends I did have had lots of problems, too; but they were true friends. In high school, I was generally accepted by the intellectual theater and music clique, and found a little company in the arts. Here, I could be a 400-pound freak and be somewhat cool. The theater thrives on extremes and drama, and that was me all over. I guess it was a form of circus sideshow, high-school style. But I never got cast in any school productions, because the teacher couldn't deal with having a 400-pound actor in any of her shows. I was relegated to backstage "technical" parts, always longing to be on the stage.

I also played the piccolo—stereotypical for a fatso, right? However, I was very good at it, eventually working so hard that I won first place in a statewide music audition for high school seniors.

What I Ate When I Was 400 Pounds

Every morning when I was still in high school, I went to a fantastic job at the local television station as a producer and director. Before I left home, I would have a huge breakfast, three or four eggs, potatoes, and a bowl of cereal—a giant version of the so-called healthy American breakfast. Then I would have a couple of doughnuts on the way to work. While at work, I would have a couple of candy bars and several Cokes for a mid-morning snack and then it'd be time for lunch and I would go to McDonald's. I remember my standard order very well: three Big Macs, two large fries, a large Coke, two apple pies, and a chocolate shake. Then I went to school.

If I made it in time, I would have another lunch at the cafeteria, then, during the day, while in class, all I'd be thinking of was how to get some more food. In my locker I kept big bags of chocolate candy with peanuts or candy bars or jellybeans. After school, I'd head to the doughnut shop and have four, five, or six doughnuts, and occasionally a couple of pieces of cake. Then I'd go off with my friends and smoke cigarettes. Just before dinner time, I'd stop again at McDonald's and have a couple of hamburgers, maybe French fries, and then I'd go home and have dinner with the family.

A "Diet" Meal, Then Ice Cream

At home, in front of my father and siblings, we would have our unpleasant diet meal.

Then, at about 8 o'clock, my mother and I would drive off, say we were going on errands, and would immediately head to the ice cream store. Every night, I would have at least three or four dips of ice cream with hot fudge sauce. Then we would drive across town and go to another ice cream store.

Often I might have the double, triple-decker, super-duper mountain-top, which was something like seven scoops of ice cream with hot fudge and nuts and whipped cream with a cherry on top, *every single evening*. I got to the point where I was unable to sleep at night unless my belly was completely filled up with ice cream. That was the typical day of a 400-pound teenager. Crazy, huh?

No Girlfriend, That's For Sure

I had a hard time as an adolescent. Most kids my age were beginning to think of the opposite sex and to be romantic and start dating. I couldn't do any of that. I did ask a few girls out, but no one would go out with me.

Imagine being a girl of normal weight, wanting to be cool and popular at school but being seen with a 400-pound guy. It just didn't work. I wanted to go to the high school prom but no one would go with me, so I simply pretended that I was above it, that it was stupid to go to the prom. In hindsight, I know it was the only choice I had. I stayed home alone that night.

I got cheated out of being a teenager because I was too fat. And I will never be a teenager again. I've learned to accept that; but for a long time it hurt. To tell you the truth, though, when I lost all this weight, I felt like I was a teenager again. I was suddenly seventeen at thirty-two years old, with a new body, a body that was useful. I could walk, I could run, I could play. It was great. I had a sex life.

Trying to Fill the Emptiness with Food

Years later I realized I had been in a lot of pain and had a lot of repressed anger. But I wasn't really aware of that at seventeen. Now I know that many people who are fat feel the emptiness I felt. When you feel empty, when you feel ashamed, when you feel that you're worthless or no good, you want to try to soothe your feelings. My way was to eat.

It's hard to feel pain. From an early age, I never wanted to feel any pain or discomfort. I didn't want to have to struggle. I had the crazy idea that everything was going to be easy and perfect. Life just isn't like that.

Until my thirties I didn't understand that pleasure was being able to live freely and fully within one's limits and boundaries, in the way our Creator intended us to be. I kept trying to be happy, kept pretending to be jolly, trying to believe that everything was fine. I could never completely feel satisfied from food. I couldn't fill the void. I was seriously, deeply hungry all the time. No amount of food in the world would fill me up. I hated my body. I couldn't walk up a flight of stairs without being totally out of breath. I couldn't stand being 400 pounds. I couldn't go to a movie theater and sit in a regular seat, so I didn't go to movies anymore. I couldn't sit in an airplane seat. I broke chairs. I couldn't walk anywhere—I had to drive or be driven. It's horrible to weigh 400 pounds. I pray to God I never weigh that much again.

I went to our family doctor and asked for some diet pills. He gave me a prescription for some strong ones, along with a poorly copied diet handout. I thought I had found the answer; now losing weight would be easy. Since I was so unhappy, I decided to make the process quicker. So I doubled the number of pills I took and began fasting. I would only have a cup of juice a day and no solid food at all. After a few weeks I got so hungry I had to eat something, so I allowed myself one can of green beans and a hamburger patty every Friday afternoon.

Mind you, I was always under supervision of my doctor. He made me come in every two weeks, get weighed by the nurse, and then spend about two minutes with me congratulating me for losing eleven to twenty pounds every week. I told him what I was eating (or wasn't) and he didn't blink an eyelid. I'd ask him for more pills, and he gladly wrote out prescription after prescription. I lost 130 pounds in only three months. And I was out of my mind, totally buzzed out from all of the diet pills. But then, on the outside, I looked great—thin and handsome! Inside, however, I was still 400 pounds: desperate, depressed, and ready to kill myself.

Right after I had lost 130 pounds, some friends of mine introduced me to Catherine Stine, a fine artist, illustrator, and painter. Actually, I was so unhappy and depressed that I was too afraid to like her at first, although I was very intrigued by her. But something inside me liked her because I started having romantic and erotic dreams with her in them! We became good friends. Then we started going out on dates and lived together for a while. After four years, we got married. I ended up gaining the weight back. Catherine still loved me anyway, even though I had a hard time loving myself. Fasting and diets, all the various programs, none of them worked. I thought I was destined to be fat forever.

I added it up recently: I've gained and lost over 1,000 pounds in my life.

A Last Resort

There was one big turning point in my life when I was thirty-two. I was smoking three packs a day; I was about 330 pounds or so. I could barely move. My wife and I weren't getting along. I hadn't worked in almost a year because nothing I tried worked, and I couldn't sell any movie or TV projects. I was a producer who was too messed up to produce. I was desperate and I knew at the core of my existence that my life had to change or I would be dead soon. I couldn't continue living the way I was living anymore. I had tried every diet and nothing had worked. I couldn't unravel the mystery of my obesity. My problems were beyond me.

People had told me that God would be there me if I ever needed help , but I always avoided that because it felt like being too weak or uncool. I'd heard about people being "saved" but thought that was corny and only for losers. While I considered myself spiritual and certainly believed in God, I felt that if I couldn't solve my own problem, then I might be better off dead. I was too proud to humble myself and admit I couldn't handle my weight problem. Until that one day, that one moment, when I just reached the end. That feeling of desperation and emptiness was too great to hold down inside anymore.

As a very final resort, I decided to go to a spiritual group meeting of people who had the same problems I did. I called the telephone number in my town and found out about that group and went. Unfortunately, there was nobody there. So I sat in a dark place in a basement meeting room all by myself, desperate and miserable. At the end of the hour, after nobody had shown up, I left. On my way out I ran into a very thin, straggly punk girl who was late for the meeting. She gave me a list of other places to go, other meetings, and other support groups.

The next morning, I went to one of them. That meeting, at a church community center, was filled with about forty people. They were mostly women, but I didn't care. It was a ninety-minute discussion group where each person spoke about how God or their "Higher Power" had helped them. At the end of the time, I was the last person who hadn't spoken and everyone looked at me.

I couldn't say a word or move an inch I was so embarrassed. After an eternity, I said to myself: "Oh my God, how am I going to get out of this?" I just burst into tears and began to tremble. The whole room was staring at me.

Then I heard words coming out of my mouth: "Well, I have this problem and I can't manage it." It wasn't *me* talking. *I* didn't know what to do. Whatever happened, the situation I now felt was out of my hands, and all I could do was just sink into the chair in a pool of emotion. Me, a fat man crying out of control… this really was the end.

But another man was there, right next to me, and he put his arm around my shoulder and said I was going to be all right. Then, all sorts of people walked over to me and hugged me and gave me little slips of paper with their phone numbers on them. I was a basket case. I couldn't believe that anyone cared about me!

A New Desire To Live

After an age of people hugging me, and being unable to say a thing, I finally quit crying and pulled myself together.

I managed to get to work, but as usual I couldn't get anything done. All I could think about was a dozen chocolate brownies at the corner bakery. I was hurting big time. My life was on the rocks. I was a fat emotional mess, an utter failure, and I had just completely embarrassed myself and let go of my pride in front of a whole crowd of strangers. Oh God, I needed relief. Those brownies were calling my name and pulling me out the door, so I got up out of my chair and went to the door. Something, however, stopped me. I think it was that desire not to die, not to eat myself into the grave. I thought about the list of steps I had heard about at that meeting. The first step was to admit I had a problem. I'd just done that. The second was to be willing to believe in something bigger than myself. I already believed in God, so that was easy. The third one was to ask God for help. That one was hard. My pride was in the way.

I thought I'd try it, nonetheless, because I was by myself in my office. There was nothing left to lose, because I'd already lost it all. I'd already embarrassed myself, already was a failure, so I didn't have to worry about failing again. I swallowed my pride, got down on my knees, and even though I thought it was humiliating, I said a prayer. Aloud, I said: "God please help me. I can't do this alone." The tears poured out of me again, this time even more uncontrollably. This time, the pain was gone. These were tears of release. This was crying for joy. Help was there, and I knew it and felt it instantly.

While I was on my knees praying, the phone rang. It was a major network calling to say they were going to give me half a million dollars to develop and produce a television movie. It was a story about Thanksgiving. I couldn't believe this was happening to me. I felt the presence of God with me, handing me a miracle. God was instantly, miraculously solving all of my problems, and all I had had to do was ask. I'll never forget that moment, and I'll never doubt the existence, helpfulness, and love of God ever again. Man, was it ever thanksgiving time!

My Show Wasn't Over, It Had Just Begun

Just as soon as I hung up the phone, the brownies were calling my name again. I began to realize that, even though God was with me, I had a choice, and it was up to me to make it. I could go to the bakery or I could go to another meeting. I decided to forgo the instant but temporary chocolate pleasure and choose long-term freedom and happiness. I decided to go to another meeting. At the back of the room was a table with all sorts of spiritual books on it. I happened to pick one up at random titled "For Today." It was one of those meditation-of-the-day calendar pocket books. I looked in that book to the day, September 6, and the thought for the day was, "God is the producer of this show, not I."

At that moment, I thought to myself: "This is another miracle happening. God is speaking to me through this book! This is no coincidence. This is God the true Producer speaking to me, reassuring me, comforting me, telling me I'm not alone. Unbelievable!"

The way was clear. All I had to do was let go and let Him be my producer. I decided then and there to do whatever it takes to let God show me the way to lose weight and get my life back.

What happened next continues to amaze me to this day. My whole being took on an ease, a kind of "rising above" perspective that let me see my life and my experiences in an entirely refreshing and peaceful way. I was no longer a product of my problems, no longer a trapped animal full of fear. I was a strong and powerful man, able to go through life without having to constantly soothe my wounds and quench my pain.

Don't get me wrong—the pain was, and is, still there. But it doesn't matter much anymore. I am now God-equipped to handle it. I'm not consumed by my eating problems, or swallowed up in fear. I no longer carry another me in fat. The deep wounds I endured are healed, for sure, but I've got a lot of scars and I don't care—I'm healed! The past really doesn't matter; now I see my scars as symbols of battles won and of survival. What's different now is that I know that I'm not a fat man out of control; I'm a whole person filled with possibilities. I am now able to look back on my life and see that I was always a good person, with a good heart and mind—it's just that my obesity problems and my swollen ego had taken the best of me and covered up all of my good parts.

This state of mind didn't just happen all at once. Living a life of joy is a process of unfolding, learning, and doing. For years I'd been reading books and taking courses in nutrition, psychology, religion, and philosophy. The recovery program I ended up devising didn't fall together with one big click: the pieces slowly fitted in with each other over several years. And I haven't finished yet! Certainly all the negative experiences I'd had were very important: the diets and pills, which are ultimately so destructive and so useless; the delibitating and self-defeating shame; the paralyzing fear. I have learned to keep letting go of that stuff, over and over, every second of every day.

I'm also happy to report that my parents also recovered from their problems, but not in a way that any of us would have preferred. My mother eventually lost some weight, but, sadly, because of a severe illness. My father did stop drinking and smoking, a major accomplishment. They both passed away too young though—victims of diseases. I'm so grateful for them, nonetheless, and I now easily forgive and appreciate them for everything they tried to do to help in their own way. I'm determined to have a better life than they did and even more dedicated to others in the same predicament I was in. Most of all, I want to help my children learn ways to be happy and not have to depend on negative habits or self-destructive behaviors for their joy. My siblings, too, have risen up from their difficult childhoods and I'm very proud of them.

In the next few pages we're going to begin your unfolding and your liberation. We're not going to wait for you to be sick or desperate any more than you may be right now. We're going to release you of your fears, shame, helplessness, and misery with High Powered help. You may not feel ready, you may still want to hold on to your troubles because you're used to them. That's OK, it happens to the best of us.

Know that I'm on your side. I offer you all my years of trial and error, and all my research and experimentation, and, honestly, my success. I can now say that I know how to lose weight and keep it off forever, because I've done it. I know how to teach you to do it too, as I have for a lot of others. You're worth it. If I can do it, so can you.

I was able to lose 160 pounds, and I am able to maintain a reasonable weight and stay healthy because I am in partnership with God. What does that mean? Simple, I make a regular effort to stay on a balanced food plan and make sure to be active every day, in exchange for God's total care and help. See, I just could never do what I wanted to do on my own. I didn't have the strength of will, or the personal fortitude or peace of mind. I was always feeling like something was missing, or that I was inferior and worthless, and unable to do what ordinary people could do. So, in desperation and pain, with a strong desire to survive and recover from my problems, I just gave up! I simply decided to just stop trying to do everything myself, and went to God for help. He was there, and was very real. (By the way, I only say "He" because that's the way the English language is constructed. I could say "She", too, but it's not what most people are used to and honestly neither gender works very well to describe our Divine Creator. God is so vast and so omnipresent, He is way beyond gender description. It is our knowledge and ability to communicate our experiences that are limited, not God.)

Once I gave my life and problems to God and asked for help, I was spiritually and emotionally released from my self-hatred enough to learn basic nutrition, healthy eating behavior, and realistic exercise. I discovered what ordinary weight people ate and how much they consumed by watching them. I took a course in food habit behavior modification. I went to nutrition classes, and read lots of books. I enrolled in the St. Luke's/Roosevelt hospital weight management program in New York City. I kept food logs for several months of everything I ate, and why, where, and how I felt while eating. I studied the USDA Food Pyramid, and then prayed for the ability to follow it. I boned-up on exercise theory and read many scientific studies. I interviewed lots of people who had lost weight and got their advice on how best to do it. I subscribed to newsletters and got lots of material from libraries on how to eat and move. What I didn't do anymore was to give my hopes away to quack fad diet books and weight loss scam products, as I did a million times in the past. I was determined to just eat and move like ordinary, everyday people, and not have to obsess, diet, or exhaust myself with strenuous exercise ever again.

With all of this effort, shortly thereafter I created my own practical eating plan, based on common sense and the USDA Food Pyramid and "Dietary Guidelines for Americans," concentrating on eating only "ones": one serving, one portion, at one time. All of the knowledge, data, and advice I'd gathered all came together for me in a profound revelation one day while walking on a quaint street in New York City's Greenwich Village, near New York University, where I went to school. I knew there was "one" God, not many, and that I was "one" person, and I'd seen that people without weight problems eat mostly "one" thing per meal, and not more than one. As this began to dawn on me, the Bob Marley song "One Love, One Heart" came wafting out of an apartment window above me. I felt a great sense of spiritual joy well up in me. The answer was simple: I should learn to eat only one serving at a time, and I should eat several small meals and snacks per day. It all came together in the Joy of Weight Loss Food and Activity Plan which has helped me and hundreds of thousands of people immensely over the last decade. And I hope it'll now help you, too.

Regarding exercise, I found out that one doesn't need to be an athlete or to slave away at intense exercise for hours a day in order to manage a weight problem. With Divine Grace I was able to get up from the couch and begin to move. It's like the fear and dread were lifted. It was truly liberating to know that just doing what I could easily do at first—about ten minutes a day of walking—would be enough. God would help me get out and do it. I was no longer alone in my problems—God was there to both show me the way and give me the strength to do what I had to do in order to be healed. In other words, there was great hope for me.

Because I felt so much happiness from God, I didn't need to stuff myself anymore. Small amounts of food were enough. I could eat anything at all, if I wanted. Having only one portion of something was truly satisfying. I no longer needed seconds or thirds to be filled. I made sure to eat from all five food groups, in exactly the amounts that the experts recommended. I stopped trying crazy diets, and got the power just to use common sense in my eating—having carbohydrates, meats and dairy, fruits and vegetables, and little or no fatty or sugary junk foods or desserts. At first I was shocked at how little food a person needs in order to live and feared that I could never survive on so little. But I knew in my soul that I needed to eat far less; so I prayed to God, and began to feel very satisfied on small amounts. From experience, I discovered how little I need to eat to be healthy. I also knew I couldn't continue to have ice cream or desserts and still lose weight, so I asked God over and over again to be free of the maddening desires.

Almost miraculously, I got that power, and my cravings were lifted. Taking it day by day, sometimes minute by minute, I just stayed on the food plan and didn't have to eat what I knew I shouldn't. I have never felt extremely hungry since, and it's been over eleven years. Now, on a non–weight loss food plan, I have absolutely anything, but am able to keep true moderation. I have desserts and occasional junk foods, and I enjoy them!

When I was still really fat, I knew I had to exercise, but I was the last person to be able to get up and do it. I absolutely positively hated to exercise. The idea of going to a gym was completely repellant. But I knew I had to do something to move my body. So I surrendered that problem to God as well. What I received was the knowledge to see it in a different light: that being just the slightest bit *active* might actually be enjoyable. That was very, very freeing to me. The knowledge that I could lose weight if I just went for a nice walk around the block every day, and that would do it, was liberating. With just that freedom, I began walking just ten minutes a day. A few months later, I discovered a stretch and easy movement class for overweight people at a nearby hospital called "Any Body Can." It was led by an angel named Joan Avalone. I prayed for God to give me the strength to go to one of the classes. Swallowing my exercise hatred, my fears and insecurities, I went. Surprise! It was actually really fun, and made me feel really good afterwards. The teacher was a sweetheart, and the other folks in it were even fatter than I was, which made me feel better about myself. I just kept doing what I'd learned: surrendering and asking for help, eating on my food plan, going for walks and to my stretch and movement group twice a week, and the weight slowly came off—about two pounds a week. Once I lost about fifty pounds, I then felt I wanted more active fun and signed up for a dance class at New York University.

I went to that class faithfully, twice a week, even though I was the only man and was out of place because I was overweight. Another really nice teacher, Abby Saxon, at first thought I was in the wrong room. But when she heard that I just wanted to learn to dance and to lose more weight she welcomed me warmly. She was a great teacher, too, making the steps easy and over-the-top fun. Great music, too. Boogie down, baby! I just love to dance! And I could do the choreography surprisingly well! I guess I was a dancer trapped in a fat man's body. I would just fly around the room and lose myself in mid-air. What joy! The weight really poured off me then—consistently two to three pounds a week. Best of all, I lost my sense of insecurity and obesity embarrassment in that class. Thank you, Abby, from the bottom of my heart.

Once I had reached a reasonable weight and kept it off for over one year, I decided I should dive into another deep fear and dread—swimming. I couldn't swim.

Remember, I told you about my horrid experiences at five years old in the swimming class? I never did go in the water after that, except once as a 400-pound teenager, and quickly sank into a lake, drowning, and had to be rescued. Me and water didn't mix, and I was terrified of it. So I followed my desire to heal that part of my past and enrolled in a beginning swimming class. Again, I was the only man in a NYU class of all Asian women! But I didn't care. I surrendered my fears and insecurities, and the teachers, Scott Wilet and Dan Cordle, taught me to swim in no time. How easy it was! How lovely to glide effortlessly through the water! What JOY! I can now swim a mile without stopping!

Another really important part of my healing process was opening myself up enough to reach out to others. The anonymous support group that I mentioned earlier was really a helpful start for me. I kept going, sometimes every day, other times once a week. I discovered that there are *lots of support groups out there*, and all I had to do was make the slightest effort to find them and just go. I love these groups. I hear great stories of other people's lives, how they lost weight and found joy and happiness, and I make a lot of new friends, too. Instantly, I found much in common with other people. I also began to make small efforts to open myself up and let others know me. I asked God to let me risk my own self-hatred and fear of embarrassment and just tell folks about my feelings, interests, experiences, needs, pains, fears, sorrows, and, most importantly, joys.

In hindsight, I'd always wished that there was one book, one source of information that had everything I needed, in a way that would actually work. With all the millions of diet and exercise books and tapes and products out there, I had never found one that had everything I needed, in the right combination of effective elements. That's why I wrote this book for you. It's my attempt to put all the pieces of the puzzle together just for you, in a way that you can actually find useful and effective. After years of trial and error, I'm grateful to God for showing me what really, truly works and to give it to you so that you will experience the freedom and joy that I have, without nearly as much work as I had to do to find it.

Today, compared to how much I hated myself as a child, I'd have to say that I'm the most "Chumley" I could be. I am perfectly imperfect. I'm a lot thinner, I'm a lot happier. Things are much lighter in my life, things are a lot easier—although life is still difficult. I've got lots to learn and a lot to accomplish. In fact, I feel that I've just begun to scratch the surface of what I'd like to do in terms of learning, service, and creativity. This book is, I hope, creative and of service to you.

I can go into any clothes shop and buy nice things right off the rack. I don't have to change my whole wardrobe over and over due to gaining and losing anymore, ever. I can wear shorts and tight-fitting tee-shirts and look good. I can dress up in a suit and tie and look like a gajillion bucks! People look at me on the streets and on the bus and subway…not because I'm fat, but because I'm thinner and handsome! I don't mind wearing a bathing suit at a public pool. I love dressing in hip, fashionable clothes and going to parties. I love dressing up for meetings and business functions. I also love just wearing old clothes and playing and getting dirty sometimes. Once, after clothes shopping one day, I was walking down a street and saw a really handsome looking man in the mirror of a storefront across the street who was wearing some really cool clothes like the ones I had just bought (and was wearing home). I looked a little closer and that handsome man in the mirror was me! Talk about joy of weight loss!

Thank you, God, for giving me my life back.

Two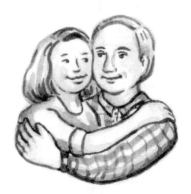

Finding and
Allowing Joy

What Is Joy?

Joy is a very glad, happy feeling. It's a radiant human emotion you get as a result of receiving pleasure, satisfaction, and comfort. Joy is a blissful experience that happens when everything in your life is fine and you are all right no matter what comes your way.

Joy is also a spiritual condition. Joy happens when you are feeling blessed. It comes when you feel the presence of your Creator, assuring you that you belong and that you're not alone. Joy is when you know you are valued and important to this great universe.

I'm sure you've experienced joy, at least a little. But you deserve a whole lot of joy, on a regular basis. Don't wait until you lose weight in order to find joy. Find and accept it now, and you will lose weight in the process. But first, be aware that you may be holding yourself back.

The key for you is to *allow joy into your life*. Starting here and now, your finding and allowing joy is our mission together. The answer you've been longing for is in turning negative and sorrowful weight loss experiences into joyous ones. Do this with God's help and you will finally be able to manage your weight (and life) problems forever. It may seem hard at first, but don't worry. I will guide you through step by step in the easiest, most effective, and quickest possible ways.

How Do You Find Joy?

- You find joy by making an effort to identify it in any given situation.

- You find joy by giving it to yourself: by doing something positive that will cause joy to happen.

- You find joy by allowing yourself to experience both joy and sorrow. To do this you surrender your blocks and fears to something bigger and more powerful than you are. (I call that something God.)

Each of us has a million different joys inside. It's simply a matter of tapping into them when you need them and creating new, positive habits of letting joy exist.

Starting now, make a constant effort to find joy in everything you do. When you work, see the positive and fruitful aspects of the job—such as the money you are paid, the help you are giving, the importance of your position. When you're taking care of personal business, find joy in getting it done as best you can. When it's time for a meal, take joy in only eating one portion. Feel the power and joy of having just enough (there's lots more on the joy of eating to come). Enjoy the good feeling of eating healthy, fresh, and nutritious food that's good for your body and mind. When you are active today, enjoy moving your body and freeing your muscles and joints. Breathe deeply the fresh air and let the rays of sunshine enter your entire being. Look at beautiful nature all around you: trees, flowers, grass, clouds, birds, and bugs—they're all gifts from God for us to enjoy.

Here are two "quick joy-starters" for you to try this moment. Pick one and do it right now:

- Close your eyes, and think of a time when you really had a good time: something like a special birthday party, a trip to a carnival or an amusement park, the moment when you just finished getting really dressed-up for a special occasion and were proud and happy with yourself. Take a moment to think of every sweet detail, all the good, joyful moments, and how wonderful you felt. If something sad comes up, fine! No problem! Let the tears flow, and go deeper and deeper into both the joy and the sorrow.

- Or think of a really special moment when you were with someone very special: a parent or family member you loved, a close friend, lover, a teacher or caregiver. It's a moment when someone really showed they loved you by something they did or gave you. Perhaps it was a time when you needed help or were in trouble; when someone reassured you or held your hand and told you everything was going to be OK. If you feel the joy mixing with sorrow and need to cry, go ahead. It's natural. Let this be a complete experience, full of emotion.

Here's a poem I wrote. It's how I find and allow joy into my life.

Joy is in release, so thankfully received.
Joy is in sorrow, so sweetly mourned and grieved,
Joy is to be found, you find it through yearning,
Joy is in coming and going, waiting and watching, living and learning.

> *If it weren't for our troubles we'd never be able to appreciate happiness.*
> —An old saying

Notice that I mentioned "joy is in sorrow." Notice, also, I mentioned sorrow in the instructions for joy and in the two jump-starts above, encouraging you to go ahead and feel it and cry if you want. This is for a reason. The secret is, that in order for joy to come in, sorrow usually has to come with it. Joy and sorrow are close friends. They are linked and cannot be separated. The same is true for pain and healing.

If you're like most of us, you've had a lot more pain and sorrow than healing and joy! It's high time you made use of those feelings. Let's now go a little deeper into the formula for joy by making good use of the sorrow and pain. After all they're there for a reason and, in that light, they may not really be so bad. Allow yourself to consider some new ideas about yourself.

A Lack of Self-Esteem

Whatever causes overweight and obesity, be it combinations of genetic, brain or body chemical imbalances, habits or conditioning, psychological or developmental problems, I'm convinced that a lack of joy and happiness due to low-self esteem and self-criticism have a lot to do with the condition. I've never met or worked with a person struggling with obesity who didn't have a rock-bottom low opinion of him- or herself somewhere in the recesses of their mind. Many have no idea they have it at all, because it's been deeply repressed for a long time.

Further, I've discovered that not only do people with substance problems (like overweight and obesity) have low self-esteem, there's often a magnified amount of sorrow and emotional pain in their lives.

A Difficult Idea To Lose

It's strange, but for some reason many of us are heavily invested in feeling bad about ourselves. We may say we want joy and happiness, but we'll actually do anything we can to avoid it. We keep on feeling inferior deep down, no matter how good we really are. We allow ourselves to tolerate too much pain and discomfort, clothes that don't fit, hampered

> *Most folks are about as happy as they make up their minds to be.*
> —Abraham Lincoln

intimacy and love-making, furniture that breaks, and poor treatment from others, swallowing our negative self-esteem over and over again. We may hate our self-hatred, but we still hold on to it underneath.

So many of us overweight people are outrageously critical of ourselves. So many of us are grandiose perfectionists and, at the same time, our worst critics. Everything we do is too hard and not good enough. Many of us feel that we're fat because we're somehow lazy, weak-willed, or inferior. How critical can you get?

This self-depreciation keeps us committing a little slow suicide with every extra bite we take, knowing full well the side-effects of eating too much. We mean well, and want to eat less and more healthily, but we need the extra comfort and fleeting pleasure of "just a little more," or "just a little sweet or high-fat food," because we hurt so badly inside. At the moment of consumption, eating in moderation seems so impossibly hard and painful that we're "unable to do it."

We avoid exercising and moving even though we know it's going to make us feel better in the long run. It's just that we can't stand any more work or any more pain— we're full up with it. We're also way overworked and overscheduled. We absolutely don't have time to commit to a regular exercise routine, and, if we did, we're just too tired and too overwhelmed to do it anyway.

Value in Misery

What would life be like if we actually did eat in moderation and get enough exercise? Would we really *like* to be healthy? What would happen if we put aside the negative thoughts and blocks? What would really happen to us if we were thinner and feeling really great?

Why can't we do what it takes to lose the weight forever? Why do we continue to eat too much and do too little physical exercise when we're unhappy? The solution seems easy enough; it just seems impossible to actually do it! It may be that the misery and suffering are actually *giving* us something. Could there be some hidden value in low self-esteem? Is there fruit in holding on to the weight?

One can spend years in therapy working on this topic. It's a big one. I do recommend therapy for people who want it and really need it—a good psychologist or pastoral care professional can be a real asset. That takes a lot of time and commitment, however. Therapy or counseling may be worth it, but there are some other, speedier ways I'd like you to consider right away.

An Inkling As To Why

So many of us hate ourselves deep down, avoid making changes, and hold on to our problems because that's what we're used to. We have lifelong investments in misery and it's really hard to put them aside. Becoming something different may be threatening and scary to our inner, unconscious mind. The way we are works well enough to get by at the moment; becoming attractive and healthy may be too much to bear. It may be upsetting the emotional apple cart to truly lose weight.

The truth is, we feel we're supposed to be in constant need and to suffer. We're supposed to hate ourselves, supposed to be fat, supposed to overeat, supposed to be sick. We've been trained to be incomplete and needy from birth. Our culture dictates it. We're supposed to be constantly hungry so we'll buy food products; we're supposed to be sickly so we'll buy medicines; we have to be fat so we can constantly purchase diet products; we're trained to feel ugly or esthetically inferior so we'll invest in fashion and cosmetics. Why do advertisers pick the most beautiful, perfect-looking people as models? So we'll feel inferior, dislike ourselves some more, and buy whatever they're selling in hopes of getting what we need. And on and on. That's one cause of low self-esteem. But there's an even deeper one.

Many parents, caregivers, and teachers inadvertently teach us to hate ourselves, in order for us to conform to society and be "normal." We were always supposed to be "good little children," the way others wanted us to be, and not the natural selves we were.

Our well-meaning adult role models may have been very critical of us. They did it in the form of "constructive criticism," so we would be more perfect and better than they are (because they felt inferior, too, perhaps). What happens when we're the target of a lot of criticism, being told we're imperfect and in need of correction over and over again? We begin to believe it. We begin to buy into the idea that we were not born normal and good, that we're grossly imperfect and need to be better, and we integrated this into our psyches at a very young age. Many well-meaning religious leaders do this too, mistakenly training us to believe we're "born sinners" or forever inferior to God. (Talk about sad!)

> *The unendurable is the beginning of the curve of joy.*
> —Djuna Barnes, Nightwood

When faced with big and powerful adult criticism, what does a little defenseless kid do? Kids haven't enough life experience yet to consider anything other than what they're told, so they believe they are inferior and need to change. They begin to make misery and inferiority their own, in order for the pain of criticism to go away. In other words, kids ultimately shut off any difficult feelings or emotional responses in order to be safe.

Some of us, from extreme cases of childhood criticism, abusive or dysfunctional families, got so much criticism and emotional pounding that we really shut down our whole personalities. We emotionally numbed ourselves, turned our uniqueness off, and became terrified of doing anything different. We learned to hate ourselves a lot, so that the adults around us would stop torturing us. It snowballed, and no matter how shut-off or deep into the shell we got, we still got hurt. Where was the relief? Where was the only easy comfort and safety? In food.

A Fat Safety Cushion

Please understand… you're not alone, and you're going to be OK—because you actually are already OK. Nearly everyone alive has some degree of sorrow, self-depreciation, or feelings of inferiority. I believe that overweight people just have a lot more of it. My personal experience and research indicates that one of the main reasons people allow themselves to be overweight is to protect themselves from the pain of living. A layer of fat around every inch of the body can act as a buffer, a kind of force-field protection zone. A body that's not so attractive can also relieve you from having to go through the ordinary pain and strain of living. In extreme cases, making yourself obese can prevent you from having to deal with intimacy and emotional needs that may be too difficult to handle at that moment, because of the past. If you're sensitive, bruised, and wounded on the inside, you need a protective layer around you.

The Bright Side

When you are joyous, look deep into your heart and you shall find it is only that which has given you sorrow that is giving you joy.

When you are sorrowful look again in your heart, and you shall see that in truth you are weeping for that which has been your delight.

—Kahlil Gibran

If you're one of us who is hurting inside, who longs for some real joy, happiness and relief—congratulations. If what I've just been talking about rings a bell, please don't worry. You're going to be freed from this insidious predicament. There's a lot of hope and potential here. The trick is to use the pain and sorrow as motivation. The secret is to allow joy and lots of powerful love into your life, so you won't have to make yourself fat or protect yourself anymore.

Allow yourself to feel every emotion you have, but in a productive way, and then let go of its power over you through spiritual and emotional surrender. Don't just shove it down and ignore it any longer! Don't just stuff your body with food in order to feel better! Use the pain and sorrow for what they're worth. It's clear God gave you your experiences in life so you can grow and learn from them.

The more you hurt, the more you'll be able to rise above it.

The more you truly want joy, the more you'll do in order to get it.

Be willing to take a leap of faith to release the hidden benefits you're getting from bad habits: safety, protection, and survival.

It's Mind Over Matter

Shift the focus. Train your mind to continually respond differently by actually acknowledging and learning to love your sorrow and emotional pain. Stop trying to banish or nullify it. You can't get rid of it—it's a part of you. Let it be there, but don't let it control you anymore. Allow that part of yourself to survive, but surrender its power over you. The next chapter is about just that.

> *Give me a dozen such heartbreaks, if that would help me to lose a couple of pounds!*
> —Colette

Allow yourself to feel the joy of living, no matter what happens! Allow yourself joy in eating good foods in moderation and in becoming active. Allow yourself a spiritual connection and a purpose in life. Always remember that from pain and sorrow, hurt and suffering, joy springs eternal.

> *I found more joy in sorrow than you could find in joy.*
> —Sara Teasdale

Find joy in the sorrow. Let joy come into your life by first accepting everything that's in you: good or bad, happy or sad. Then allow that joy to grow in you by slowly feeling the sadness and sorrow, accepting the self-criticism, doubt, shame, and worry as being a complete part of you and something you can deal with. It's now OK to try something new.

Here we go together into new frontiers of your life. You're ready to allow yourself some lasting joy and freedom, finally, and it is through God's grace that you'll now receive it.

PSALM 36

7 How excellent is thy loving kindness, O God! therefore the children of men put their trust under the shadow of thy wings.

8 They shall be abundantly satisfied with the fatness of thy house: and thou shalt make them drink of the river of thy pleasures.

9 For with thee is the fountain of life: in thy light shall we see light.

Three

The Joy Of Weight Loss Personal Program

Part I: THE JOY OF SURRENDER

> *God offers to every mind its choice between truth and repose. Take which you please; you can never have both.*
>
> —Ralph Waldo Emerson

What I'm encouraging you to do may seem difficult at first but will prove to be the simplest and most effective way to relieve all your suffering and find deep and lasting joy.

I'm suggesting that you give a gift to your creator. Give the gift of all your problems. Put aside your temporary pleasures of too much food, too much leisure, and inactivity. Let go of your many thoughts of self-hatred and fear. Let go of your ego that's getting in the way of your salvation from obesity. I'm suggesting you give up your troubles, quit fighting, and trade them in for something better. Give up the past and all of your mistaken attempts, as well as the sorrow and pain. Let go of the constant self-pleasuring in order to gain something much better—infinite peace and happiness in the arms of your creator, God.

There is such safety, peace, and joy with God: a loving presence, a deep calm of great reassurance. God is available to you always, twenty-four hours a day, seven days a week, 366 days a year. And you don't have to use public transportation to find Him, either!

The truth is that God is ready for you. You are already with God; you are just avoiding Him. All that needs to be done is to acknowledge God and finally receive His gift of love.

Get out of your own way, open your eyes, and see God. Open your heart and feel His presence. Let go of the past and go into the future with God, together.

In other words: Discover and let yourself experience the secret that will completely solve your weight problems and all of your problems. The way to receive genuine freedom from the tyranny of your old, self-defeating behaviors is....

ASK GOD FOR HELP.

Keep reading. Don't stop here! We're going to do it together, with an elegant and simple method in the next few pages. It's a memorable, private ritual between you and God that you'll never forget.

I ask you: Do you put your faith or spiritual practice truly into your life experience? Do you ask God for help with everything? Or do you think yourself unworthy, or guilty, or a sinner? Perhaps you only feel worthy of God's help when you're in a severe crisis or life-threatening situation. (Be real: This is one of those times. Obesity is a health crisis, and so is an unhappy life.)

Let's start by thinking of a few instances of when God has helped you. Have you ever had a "visitation," or "spiritual awakening?" Have you ever experienced God directly? Perhaps you sometimes feel the presence of a guardian angel or a saint, caring for you from above. Maybe you've felt the divine hand of a master—like Jesus, the Buddha, Moses, Mohammed, Krishna, or a guru. Maybe you were in an accident and were saved, or you couldn't figure your way out of a crisis and suddenly God was there and showed you the way. But you don't need a crisis to experience God: All you need is to do what He wants you to do. Just get in-sync with Him and your life and your weight will become manageable again. After all, He created you. You are His child. God, the best father of all, loves His children and will not let you down, ever.

> *God's grace is the beginning, the middle, and the end. When you pray for God's grace, you are like someone standing neck-deep in water and yet crying for water. It is like saying that someone neck-deep in water feels thirsty, or that a fish in water feels thirsty, or that water feels thirsty.*
>
> —Ramana Maharshi

Many people are embarrassed to ask God to help them with their weight problems (or anything else, for that matter). Many are ashamed to admit that they have a problem at all and need help. Many even think that God is some huge thing up in the heavens, unavailable, scrutinizing your every move, some old mean man to be feared.

Is that you?

The truth is that God isn't *only* "out there," or "up there," some "bigger Higher Power." He's also "in there," inside you, looking through you, making you, breathing you, living you, loving you. Truth is, God is everywhere and in everything. It's impossible to be outside of Him. God is so vast and all powerful, so totally present, that it is very easy to miss seeing Him—and fall into the illusion that all there is is what we, alone, perceive. But the answer, again, is very simple: plain as the nose on your face! All it takes is for you to put yourself aside and allow yourself to see Him and make yourself available to Him, by asking for His help.

This isn't just faith. This is experience. God already knows you. Now, know Him.

The great Russian novelist Leo Tolstoy puts the reality of God's all pervasive existence beautifully in his description of the moment when he asked God for help, just as you're about to do....

I remember one day in early spring, I was alone in the forest, lending my ear to its mysterious noises. I listened, and my thought went back to what for these three years it always was busy with—the question of God. But the idea of him, I said, how did I ever come by the idea?

And again there arose in me, with this thought, glad aspirations towards life. Everything in me awoke and received a meaning... why do I look farther? A voice within me asked. He is there: he, without whom one cannot live. To acknowledge God and to live are one in the same thing. God is what life is. Well, then! Live, seek God, and there will be no life without him....

After this, things cleared up within me and about me better than ever, and the light has never wholly died away. I was saved from suicide.

That little voice inside him asked, "Why do I look farther?" God was already there. All Tolstoy had to do was open himself up and listen. God then revealed Himself. It's like noticing for the first time you have toes and realizing that without them you could never have walked!

Here's another radiantly shining story of a young boy, Jacques Lusseyran, blinded by a horrible accident when he was only seven years old. Ordinarily, one would think that such a event would ruin someone's life, but for Lusseyran it was the dawning of a whole new vision. With a new set of spiritual eyes.

(A few weeks after the accident) I still wanted to use my eyes. I followed their usual path. I looked in the direction where I was in the habit of seeing before the accident.... Finally, I realized that I was looking in the wrong way. I was looking too far off, and too much on the surface of things.... I began to look more closely, not at things but at a world closer to myself, looking from an inner place to one further within, instead of clinging to the movement of sight toward the world outside. Immediately the substance of the universe drew together, redefined and peopled itself anew. I was aware of a radiance emanating from a place I knew nothing about, a place, which might as well have been outside me as within.... I felt indescribable relief, and happiness so great it almost made me laugh.... Sighted people always talk about the night of blindness, and that seems to them quite natural. But there is no such night, for at every waking hour and even in my dreams I lived in a stream of light.

Sometimes it takes choosing to look in other directions, for other answers that you haven't tried or didn't want to face, to see your situation in a different light. Unfortunately, you don't always have a choice. Many times it takes something far more difficult—an accident, or severe misfortune, or losing something very precious—to force you to look to God inside you and seek God's help, because there's nowhere else to turn.

This is exactly what happened to a young, very rich, and wildly successful Wall Street businessman in the 1920s called Bill W. As he made more and more money on his investments, Bill became obsessed with seeking as much pleasure as he could from

EXODUS (HOLY BIBLE / TORAH)

3: 13 Moses said to God, "When I come to the Israelites and say to them 'The God of your fathers has sent me to you,' and they ask me 'What is His name?' what shall I say to them?"

3: 14 And God said to Moses, "Ehyeh-Asher-Ehyeh" (translated: "I Am That I Am"). He continued, "Thus shall you say to the Israelites, 'Ehyeh' ("I Am") sent me to you.'"

alcohol. He would spend all day and night drinking, never caring that he was losing his friends, his business, and his marriage with every tilt of the glass. He thought he knew everything and could control his own life. Then, on that fateful day in October 1929 his world came crashing down and he lost everything he had. For five years he barely scraped by with a bunch of menial jobs, only to quickly lose them because of his drinking. In and out of hospitals, he would sober up for a time but then quickly return to the temporary pleasures and false safety of gin. One day, however, a friend called— a real friend, who had experienced a miracle, a fellow alcoholic who, like Bill W., had nowhere else to turn, and had found a spiritual solution that truly works: admitting your problems, giving up, and asking God for help. The rest is legendary. Bill W. went on to co-found Alcoholics Anonymous.

Bill W. was a man who had always believed in some kind of universal energy, force, or higher power, but he left it to people far more religious than he to put belief into action. He was irritated by ministers and clergy.

The friend who came to visit had been helped by God. He told Bill that he, too, could not solve his own substance problems—they were too big for him to handle alone. Doctors couldn't help, his willpower was weak, and he was about to be locked up in a court-ordered drunk-tank. He had admitted complete failure, asked God for help, and ever since his whole life had turned around. It was as if the problem was lifted, almost magically, forever.

Hearing his friend's profound relief, Bill began to see another way of being. He realized that he was powerless, too, and he began to want God. His beliefs became real the moment he put himself and his problems aside and humbly asked God to help.

Instantly, Bill felt a kind of calm and profound relief. His insane desire for alcoholic anesthesia was immediately lifted. He was able to have his life back—but this time, it was a new, easier life without a ton of self-hindering fears and worries. He no longer needed self-anesthesia.

Whether your experience is instant or takes a lifetime, God's presence and help is there, immediately for the asking. If you need proof, just look at the millions and millions of recovered alcoholics who have been helped by God through the AA Twelve-Step program of recovery. The program has been translated into every language and applied to virtually every other addiction as well, because it works. God works. I recommend Overeaters Anonymous, a Twelve-Step program for food addictions and compulsive overeating. Every town and city has regular meetings: they're in the phone book. OA doesn't cost money and you'll find support and encouragement from people like me, who have recovered from obesity and want to share our spiritual liberation with others. You'll meet friends there—people who understand because they've been where you are.

Your spiritual recovery may happen in a miraculous enlightenment as it did for Bill W., after decades of self-destruction. Or it may be subtle or come in ways you least expect. It's up to God. One thing for sure, you have to find the desire in you and work towards being open and willing. Everyone does it differently; there's no one-size-fits-all approach.

You can come to God from any religion or spiritual practice. You can use any sage, savior, or saint. Or you can just go directly, easily, just by asking—we'll do it together shortly. Although religions are different, of course, with different beliefs and methods, at the heart they're all saying the same thing—God (your Creator) is there for you, available, inside you. There are different names for God, sure. There are different words, languages, customs, rituals, tenets—and nearly every religion strongly believes that it is the only true way. But the truth is, God is non-denominational.

A difficult but very fruitful way to go to God for help is to realize that you're in trouble. Let your suffering and sorrow really motivate you. Let your failed attempts at dieting and humiliating, fruitless resolutions, as well as a gigantic desire to just "give up," guide you forward toward surrendering. Perhaps realizing that you are not living well will motivate you finally to give your problems and your life to God. This is what happened to David Brainerd (1718–1747) an American protestant missionary. A very emotional and sickly child, Brainerd achieved a religious conversion and saw the Christ Spirit within him, after much anguish, in 1739.

> I was walking again, in a solitary place, in a mournful melancholy state. I was attempting to pray; but found no heart to engage in that or any other duty; my former concern, exercise, and religious affections were now gone. I thought that the Spirit of God had quite left me; but still was not distressed; yet disconsolate, as if there was nothing in heaven or earth could make me happy. Having been thus endeavored to pray—though, as I thought, very stupid and senseless—for near half an hour; then as I was walking in a thick grove, unspeakable glory seemed to open to the apprehension of my soul. I do not mean any external brightness, nor any imagination of a body of light, but it was a new inward apprehension or view that I had of God, such as I never had before, nor

anything which has the least resemblance to it. I had no particular apprehension of any one person in the Trinity, either the Father, the Son, or the Holy Ghost; but it appeared to be Divine glory. My soul rejoiced with joy unspeakable, to see such a God, such a glorious Divine Being; and I was inwardly pleased and satisfied that he should be God over all for ever and ever. My soul was so captivated and delighted with the excellency of God that I was even swallowed up in him; at least to that degree that I had no thought about my own salvation, and scarce reflected that there was such a creature as myself. I continued in this state of inward joy, peace, and astonishment, till near dark without any sensible abatement; and then began to think and examine what I had seen; and felt sweetly composed in my mind all the evening following. I felt myself in a new world, and everything about me appeared with a different aspect from what it was wont to do. At this time, the way of salvation opened to me with such infinite wisdom, suitableness, and excellency, that I wondered I should ever think of any other way of salvation; was amazed that I had not dropped my own contrivances, and complied with this lovely, blessed and excellent way before. If I could have been saved by my own duties or any other way that I had formerly contrived, my whole soul would now have refused it. I wondered that all the whole did not see and comply with this way of salvation, entirely by the righteousness of Christ.

Inward experiences of God are intensely beautiful! I encourage you to have one yourself! Muhammad Ali, the famous boxer who entertained and impressed millions of fans, experienced God and converted to Islam after seeing millions of people in prayer:

> I have had many nice moments in my life. But the feelings I had while standing on Mount Arafat (just outside Mecca, Saudi Arabia) on the day of the Hajj (the Muslim pilgrimage), were the most unique. I felt exalted by the indescribable spiritual atmosphere there as over one and a half million pilgrims invoked God to forgive them for their sins and bestow on them His choicest blessings.
>
> It was an exhilarating experience to see people belonging to different colors, races and nationalities, kings, heads of state, and ordinary men from very poor countries all clad in two simple white sheets praying to God without any sense of either pride or inferiority. It was a practical manifestation of the concept of equality in Islam.

The experience of God transcends anything you've ever known. Use your spiritual or religious practices to lead you to the door. Use your love and desire to walk through it.

Getting Help To Ask For Help

God is ready. He's always been there; you've just been under the illusion that it was only you. This is the real cause of your suffering. You are just waking up to this illusion. You've thought that you were all there is. You've thought that living your life was all up to you. You thought you had to do everything by yourself: make money, get and keep a house, take care of yourself (and others), and give yourself pleasures. These necessities were, and are, a great burden. You feel you can barely hold it all together, sometimes. You've needed comfort and pleasure. You've gotten into the habit of resorting to the easiest method of comfort and pleasure there is—food. Instead of facing the pain and hardship of life directly, you've buffered it with extra servings, sweets, and snacks. It was, for the moment, easier. Yet, now it's a habit that controls you. Instead of feeling the magnificent presence of God—of life itself—in you, you've settled for less. You've compromised with external possessions and temporary pleasures, instead of allowing yourself to achieve true, infinite spiritual happiness.

Don't get me wrong—I'm not saying you were not supposed to do that, or that you were wrong. All I'm saying is that now there is a new, better, non-destructive way of finding joy and ultimate happiness in life.

And all you need to do is be willing to see that there is more to your life, than just you, alone. All you need to do to end this seemingly endless cycle of suffering/pleasuring and pleasuring/suffering is to ask God for help.

You know it. You know you need God. You want to find permanent happiness and live it forever. But perhaps it's impossibly difficult for you to just admit you're causing your own pain and suffering, and surrender them to God. The habits and pain make you feel alive. You think it might be too hard to handle being healthy and well! And it is, without God's help!

Right now, it might be too hard to handle facing God directly inside yourself. If this is so, then I suggest asking for help, in order to ask for help. There are many helpers available who can help you go directly to God. Avail yourself of a teacher, preacher, savior, saint, guru, imam, or guardian angel. Try Jesus, Moses, Muhammad, Krishna, or Buddha if you wish. Choose a helper you can really

> *The feeling for the infinite… can be attained only if we are bounded to the utmost. The greatest limitation for man is the "self"; it is manifested in the experience: "I am only that!"*
>
> —Carl Jung

trust, someone who will lovingly guide you to God. That's the true test—if the helper shows you the way to God. (Be careful, there are those who will pretend to help you find God, but they're really only in it for themselves. These are the false prophets who are in it only for their profits.)

I want to share with you another amazing story of how an ordinary guy, a Christian, who was deeply trapped in bad habits of promiscuous sex and drinking, but had always believed in God and wanted to find him, actually did. He got help, just like you can. He was helped by an angel, who guided him to God in a miraculous way. He, too, was addicted to pleasure; his mind was split between habit and spiritual desire, too... but, with God's help, he overcame his pain and suffering forever, and later became a saint. St. Augustine tells his story:

> I longed to [devote myself to God] but I was held fast not in fetters clamped upon me by another, but by my own will which had the strength of iron chains. The enemy held my will in his power and from it he had made a chain and shackled me. For my will was perverse and lust had grown from it, and when I gave in to lust habit was born, and when I did not resist the habit it became a necessity....These two wills within me, one old, one new, one the servant of the flesh, the other of the spirit, were in conflict and between them they tore my soul apart.
>
> ...I was in torment, reproaching myself more bitterly than ever as I twisted and turned in my chain. . . . All the same it held me. And you, O Lord, never ceased to watch over my secret heart. . . . I kept saying "Let it be now, let it be now!", and merely by saying this I was on the point of making it, but I did not succeed.
>
> I was held back by mere trifles, the most paltry inanities, all my old attachments. They plucked at my garment of flesh and whispered, "Are you going to dismiss us? From this moment we shall never be with you again, forever and ever. From this moment you will never again be allowed to do this thing or that, for evermore." . . . Habit was too strong for me when it asked "Do you think you can live without these things?"
>
> ...I probed the hidden depths of my soul and wrung its pitiful secrets from it, and when I mustered them before the eyes of my heart, a great storm broke within me, bringing with it a great deluge of tears....For I felt that I was still the captive of my sins, and in my misery I kept crying "How long shall I go on saying

'tomorrow, tomorrow'? Why not now? Why not make an end of my ugly sins at this moment?"

I was asking myself these questions, weeping all the while with the most bitter sorrow in my heart, when all at once I heard the singing voice of a child in a nearby house. Whether it was the voice of a boy or a girl I cannot say, but again and again it repeated the refrain "Take it and read, take it and read."... I stemmed my flood of tears and stood up, telling myself that this could only be a divine command to open my book of Scripture and read the first passage on which my eyes should fall.... I seized it and opened it, and in silence I read the first passage on which my eyes fell: Not in reveling and drunkenness, not in lust and wantonness, not in quarrels and rivalries. Rather, arm yourselves with the Lord Jesus Christ; spend no more thought on nature and nature's appetites. (Rom. 13:13,14.) I had no wish to read more and no need to do so. For in an instant, as I came to the end of the sentence, it was as though the light of confidence flooded into my heart and all the darkness of doubt was dispelled.

Take Joy in Surrendering

Now, I encourage you to allow yourself a miracle.

Make a personal, private spiritual ritual, in a special place.

This is your secret, private act—your gift of Love. No one needs to know about it, except your creator.

Today, at your earliest opportunity before this day is over, take yourself to a special and memorable place where you can be alone. This may be your city apartment or home. A room upstairs, or in a basement where you can close the door and have an inner sanctum away from anyone else. It might be your place of worship: a church, temple, synagogue, a little side chapel or prayer lodge. You might find sanctuary in nature: a park, forest, nature preserve, garden or arboretum, or a beautiful cemetery. Just find a place where you can be by yourself, where no one will see you or make you feel self-conscious (more than you probably already are!). Go to a place that's serene and comfortable, a place you love. Any special place where you can be alone with God. (You only need fifteen minutes; longer if you wish.)

Get comfortable. Close your eyes and be silent.

Just for a moment. Be completely still in body, and mind. Let all of your thoughts melt away like ice melting into water and then flow out of you into the ground. When a thought comes up, don't go with it or cling to it. Let it float away like a cloud in a brisk wind. Do this for a minute or two, enough time to lightly clear your mind.

Don't worry that you find this difficult, everyone does. The point is simply to learn to let thoughts go by without clinging to them, not to eliminate all thoughts (that's impossible!).

> *God, whose love and joy are present everywhere, can't come to visit you unless you aren't there.*
> —Angelus Silesius

Make a personal, private prayer.

Now form a little prayer in your own words asking God for help. It could be something like:

"God, I need your help with my weight problem. I can't do it alone any more. I surrender." *or:* "God, please show me what you want me to weigh, and how to maintain it. I'm willing." *or:* "I love you, God. I need you. Please guide me to a healthy, happy life."

> *Prayer doesn't change God, but changes him who prays.*
> —Søren Kierkegaard

Lower your head to the ground.

Now, get down on your knees, and then lower your forehead to the ground. Or you could, even better, lie completely face down. Let all of your muscles relax. Release everything, let it flow into the ground and into God's hands. (If you have physical problems, simply bow your head while seated. It's the good intention that matters.) This is a marvelously powerful technique practiced for thousands of years by billions of people. All religions have their variations on this physical act, because it works. It helps you really get humble, because your body and mind are connected, and when your body surrenders your mind more easily follows.

Ask God for help.

Now, say your private prayer to God both inwardly and out loud, surrendering all of your problems and sincerely asking for help.

If you've chosen to work with a spiritual master or guide, ask them to give you the strength right now to talk to God directly. Put all hesitations aside and just do it.

Continue a patient, silent meditation.

Stay on the ground for a little while, totally quiet and empty of all expectations and hopes. Forget everything you've learned for a moment. Remember, this is a gift you're giving to God: a gift of yourself. If you're full of desire for a return, or expect things to happen in a certain way, that's your own ego trying to control God. Picture yourself as an empty container. Just be quiet and empty.

Now, pick yourself up and be seated. Close your eyes again, and be silent a little while longer. God is there when everything else disappears. Relax, He will show himself when you least expect it, and in His own special way. It's not up to you anymore.

> *PSALM 23*
> *1 The Lord is my shepherd; I shall not want.*
> *2 He maketh me to lie down in green pastures: he leadeth me beside the still waters.*
> *3 He restoreth my soul: he leadeth me in the paths of righteousness for his name's sake.*
> *4 Yea, though I walk through the valley of the shadow of death, I will fear no evil: for thou art with me; thy rod and thy staff they comfort me.*
> *5 Thou preparest a table before me in the presence of mine enemies: thou anointest my head with oil: my cup runneth over.*
> *6 Surely goodness and mercy shall follow me all the days of my life: and I will dwell in the house of the Lord for ever.*

People I have known and worked with over the years have all had individual, personal experiences of God. God delights us uniquely. For some it's an amazing transformation. Others don't realize anything different at first but slowly begin to see God's presence and work in very subtle and numerous ways. If you do not instantly feel anything different... just wait... you will!

> *If your desire lies open to God, who is your Father and sees in secret, He will answer you. For the desire of your heart is itself your prayer...Therefore, if you wish to pray without ceasing, do not cease to desire .... It never ceases to sound in the hearing of God.*
> —*Saint Augustine (354–430), On Psalm 37*

Repeat this moment again and again.

Don't forget, good things come to those who wait. Be patient. And do it again and again.

Whenever you need help, remember this moment, this gift you gave, and give it again. You can do it on your knees or just picture your surrendering in your mind. You now have a very powerful experience, the pivotal moment in your life when you gave up and asked God for assistance. Now that you did it the first time, doing so again is easier and easier. You'll get to the point where you love doing this so much and it's so much a part of you, you cannot wait to do it again—because it's wonderfully pleasurable! Loving God, loving you.

You can again give this gift of love to God, anytime, anywhere. For a split second just imagine yourself bowing down, surrendering, loving Him, asking for help. It's especially powerful when you do this in your greatest time of need—like when you're about to compulsively overeat. Or when you know you shouldn't do what you are about to do, and can't control it yourself. Ask God for the power to do the right thing. And let God take care of you, and the problem.

PSALM 16

1 Preserve me, O God: for in thee do I Put my trust.

9 Therefore my heart is glad, and my glory rejoiceth: my flesh also shall rest in hope.

11 Thou wilt shew me the path of life: in thy presence is fullness of joy; at thy right hand there are pleasures for evermore.

Enjoy and Use The Gifts That God Gives You

Think of how God has already given you the gifts of health and life. Think of how you are able to walk, run, play, and move. Think about the fact that you have an abundance of food to be able to overeat while millions in this world are starving. Think about your ability to think! Every day, every second that you choose to remain unhealthy, obese, and unfit you are shortening your own life and rejecting the greatest gifts that God has already given you. You need to realize that you are making yourself miserable and unhealthy by denying God. There's absolutely no reason to suffer this problem for one more second. Keep asking God for help, over and over again. Do it now if you didn't already!

It's an odd paradox, but it's true: the more you give of yourself to God, with no thought of return, the more He gives you in return. Everything is taken care of. I can't explain it. Just experience it for yourself. Trust your whole life to Him. Give 100 percent of your life to God and everything becomes right, beyond your wildest dreams. You find supreme happiness and never need to satisfy yourself with too much food, drink, laziness, or lethargy ever again. You become a perfect manifestation of God, the way He designed you. You don't need faith after a while, because you have real proof. You become completely convinced!

The Holy Qu'ran:
SECTION 6.
53. Say: "O my Servants who Have transgressed against their souls!
Despair not of the Mercy of Allah: for Allah forgives
All sins: for He is Oft-Forgiving, Most Merciful."

You Are Forgiven By God

Now that you have asked for God's help, and are allowing yourself to receive it, there's an added bonus: Forgiveness. God will not only help you every time you need it, whenever you ask, He can also relieve you of your past mistakes and any guilt you bear for making them. Just ask. You are meant to be here, to be human, to live your life to the fullest extent with God's permission or He would not have made you and you would not be here!

Divine forgiveness and the lasting solutions to your weight and life problems will be yours through:

- Repeated prayers, asking God for help.

- Making a regular effort to find joy, eating healthily, and being active.

- Continual acknowledgement and appreciation of God in every way possible.

If you will give these three gifts to yourself and to God you will begin to experience the joy of weight loss and infinite happiness.

Part II: EAT HEALTHILY AND BE ACTIVE

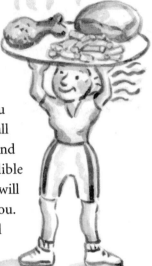

You've done the groundwork: finding joy and allowing yourself to experience it in whatever way it comes, then surrendering your problems and asking God for help. The efforts you have made so far will guide you well. Allowing yourself to feel all your emotions, happy or sad, and tapping into the incredible spiritual well of God's grace will constantly let joy grow in you. This joy and happiness will motivate you to alter your eating and moving habits day by day, for the rest of your life, and the effort itself will also be a joy. Keep up the good work!

> *Regard thy table as the table before the Lord. Chew well, and hurry not.*
>
> —Zohar (13th century AD Jewish mystical writings)

In the National Weight Control Registry project, the largest study of successful weight maintenance yet, "89% of the participants reported modifying both dietary intake and physical activity levels to achieve their successful weight loss."

Yes, be relieved! You're about to feel really great for the rest of your life! The pleasure of personal change taking place, old habits falling away, and your consistent openness and surrender to a new lifestyle will increase joy inside you tenfold every day, every moment. This joy will now, wondrously, spark your fire of desire to naturally choose healthier foods in smaller amounts. You'll also want to increase your physical and emotional joy by moving and being active every day. Eating less food will make your mind clearer and more focused. Being active will give you even more clarity, help with any depression you may have,

> *There is no sincerer love than the love of food.*
>
> —George Bernard Shaw

and fill you with vital energy. You're already started; things will only get better from now on.

Now that you're with God, you will find that He is always there guiding you, inspiring you, making things happen right. You're now in a partnership with God. All you have to do is be willing, ask for guidance, and follow His lead—making a consistent effort to be your best. Everything will fall into place, you'll have no worries or fears!

We will now devote some time and attention to what healthy eating in moderation and being active can mean for you. We'll make an effort to learn the basics of what and how much you should eat and do every day. You will begin to feel real, lasting joy and the freedom to eat whatever you like—never being chained to a deprivation diet ever again. You will feel the joy of eating only as much as you need—never overeating again and never feeling shameful or guilty about your food consumption. Starting now, you will want to move your body and be moderately active—because it brings you joy and makes you feel good and alive again, better than ever before.

Be Free of Dieting and Intense Exercise

Where most people trying to lose weight go wrong is that they try to change years of poor habits all at once. They think that the problem is only about food and overeating. Many of us have resorted to drastic, mistaken methods of dieting that restrict types of foods and make us eat only extremely low-calorie or low-fat foods. Many current diets tell us to combine "magic foods" to put our body into various states of dietary shock. Sure we lose weight at first, but it doesn't last because we can't keep it up. There's no joy in those attempts; they're too radical to integrate into our lifestyle. Other diets are just the opposite—they tell us that we can eat anything we want, as much as we want and, by taking a pill or just simply loving ourselves more,

Obesity treatment programs that rely solely on diets, especially those that are severely restrictive in regard to choices, have poor long-term outcomes; within two or three years most dieters regain all of the weight they lost.

we'll lose weight. Those attempts don't work either, because there's no structure, no shift in thinking or habits. A food addict without limits will never be able to know how much is enough or too much, and doesn't have the personal will-power to stop. Pills always have nasty side effects. These plans I call "one-dimensional," because they only address one part of the whole picture—and that is food. Being overweight or obese is a multidimensional problem.

That's all over, thank God. The past is in the past. What you're about to learn is simple common sense, practical truth, and sensible structure.

Read this chapter and let the ideas percolate in you. When it comes time for you to start making changes, I recommend following Chapter 5, The Joy of Weight Loss Daily Companion, which will slowly guide you well.

A Common Sense Method That Can Work For You

The eating plans you're about to learn are a way to always eat the right amount of a healthy range of foods for you. With a little practice, it will easily become second nature. You will not be hungry, because you'll be eating food throughout the day. You will never feel deprived, because you have the freedom to eat absolutely anything you choose. You will feel a lot of joy because, with freedom of choice practice and some basic nutritional education, you'll begin to instinctively eat what's right for you. You'll feel noticeably better soon and the weight will slowly come off. I developed these plans from years of trial and error and from a lot of studying. It works, and works so well you'll never want to eat any other way again.

> *One cannot think well, love well, sleep well, if one has not dined well.*
> —Virginia Woolf

Rest assured that these eating plans are rational and full of common sense, because they are based on the USDA Food Pyramid and the Food Guidelines for Americans. I've crosschecked their minimum recommendations and made them really easy to follow within whichever structured Joy of Weight Loss eating schedule you choose.

The USDA Food Guide Pyramid was created by teams of top professionals and has been used by hundreds of millions of people. If you follow this food plan exactly, you can get the nutrients you need, naturally eat less, and slowly lose excess weight and maintain it at the most reasonable point that God, you, a nutritionist, or registered dietician and your doctor will all agree with.

Eat Well, and Be Liberated

I believe in just eating and being free to eat whatever one likes within a structured food plan—but being completely liberated from compulsive overeating, and always eating in a healthy way in moderation. I never knew what moderation meant. I had to learn it. I weighed and measured, carried calorie and fat counters around forever and a day, took classes in nutrition and behavior modification, and got completely overwhelmed and didn't follow it all anyway when it came time to eat!

So I developed two really easy and sensible plans to eat in a normal, healthy way, still having the freedom to eat what I wanted. I distilled tons of food research into a few short pages of essential information. I share it with you right now. All you need to know about food is contained here. Just learn the following few points—the eating plan, the USDA Food Pyramid food groups and general serving sizes—and you're on your way to permanent weight management and a lot of joy.

There are two Joy of Weight Loss Eating plans: one for eating small portions of main meals and snacks, six times a day, and one where your eat three larger meals, and limit snacks. Pick either one, or try one on some days and the other the rest of the time. No matter which way you choose to eat through any given day—the point is to eat the minimum number of servings from all six USDA Food Pyramid Food Groups in any given day.

Some words of caution, however. If you are pregnant or nursing, or if you have any diseases or health problems it is essential that you consult your physician before making any significant changes in your eating habits or physical activities to ensure that what you propose for yourself is nutritionally sound, safe, and healthy.

The Joy of Weight Loss Eating Plan
Three Meals/Three Snacks a Day

This is the main recommended plan. Choose this plan if you like to eat small amounts all day long.

- Start with silence each time you eat, in recognition and appreciation of God, the food, and your healthy efforts.

- Make eating joyful and pleasurable, in moderation.

- Eat the following recommend servings in one day from all six USDA Food Guide Pyramid food groups:*

GRAINS GROUP: six servings/day (one serving = 1 slice bread or 1 oz. cereal, $\frac{1}{2}$ cup rice or pasta)*

VEGETABLE GROUP: three servings/day (one serving = $\frac{1}{2}$ cup cooked or 1 cup raw leafy, or $\frac{3}{4}$ cup juice)*

FRUIT GROUP: two servings/day (one serving = one medium fruit or $\frac{1}{2}$ cup chopped/cooked, or $\frac{3}{4}$ cup juice)*

MEAT/FISH/BEANS/NUTS GROUP (Proteins): two servings/day (one serving= two or three ounces cooked lean meat or $\frac{1}{3}$ cup cooked beans, or 2 tbs. nut butter, or $\frac{1}{3}$ cup)*

DAIRY GROUP (Proteins): two servings/day (one cup milk or yogurt or 1.5 ounces natural cheese, or two ounces processed cheese)*

FATS, OILS, SWEET GROUP: limit these foods, choose lower fat foods with no added sugars

- For a snack of if you're still hungry have one serving of a vegetable and/or a fruit.

- Be sure to always eat in balance: having a protein, grain, and fruit or vegetable each meal....

Eat Three Meals Per Day

consisting of at least *one serving from three of the USDA Food Pyramid food groups**

PROTEIN: choose either one serving from the meat/fish/beans/nuts group or one serving from the Dairy group each meal. Alternate between the two groups for each meal.*

GRAIN: one serving from the Bread, Cereal, Rice or Pasta group*

FRUIT OR VEGETABLE: one serving from either group. Alternate between the two groups for each meal.*

Eat Three Snacks Per Day

consisting of at least *one serving from three of the USDA Food Pyramid food groups**

GRAIN: one serving from the bread, cereal, rice or pasta group*

FRUIT OR VEGETABLE: one serving from either group. Alternate between the two groups for each snack.*

PROTEIN: choose either one serving from the meat/fish/beans/nuts group or one serving from the dairy group each meal. Alternate between the two groups for each snack.*

- **DRINK six glasses of water a day (eight to ten ounces each).**

- **WAIT twenty minutes after each meal to feel full.**

- **EAT VERY SLOWLY. STOP after eating everything on your day's plan. Ask God for help every time.**

*USDA Food Pyramid serving sizes are minimums for most women and older adults. If you are a teenage boy or very active person (thirty or more minutes/day) you may need more servings. Consult with your doctor or dietician/nutritionist to set the right amount to lose between a half and two pounds per week. This plan is not for pregnant or nursing women.

From the book *The Joy of Weight Loss* by Norris Chumley, published by Lantern Books, 2001. Copyright and Trademark 2001 by Norris J. Chumley. All Rights Reserved.

The Joy of Weight Loss Eating Plan
—3 Meals a Day

Choose this alternate plan if you want to eat larger meals.

- Start each meal with silence, in recognition and appreciation of God, the food, and your healthy efforts.

- Make eating joyful and pleasurable, in moderation.

- Eat the following recommend servings in one day from all six **USDA Food Guide Pyramid food groups:***

GRAINS GROUP: six servings/day, preferably whole grains (one serving = one slice bread or one oz. cereal, 1/2 cup rice or pasta)*

VEGETABLES GROUP: three servings/day (one serving = 1/2 cup cooked or one cup raw/leafy, or 3/4 cup juice)*

FRUIT GROUP: two servings/day (one serving = one medium fruit or 1/2 cup chopped/cooked, or 3/4 cup juice)*

MEAT/FISH/BEANS/NUTS GROUP (Proteins): two servings/day (one serving = two to three ozs. cooked lean meat or 1/3 cup cooked beans, or two tbs. nut butter, or 1/3 cup nuts)*

DAIRY GROUP (Proteins): two servings/day (one cup milk or yogurt or 1.5 ozs. natural cheese, or two ozs. processed cheese)*

FATS, OILS, SWEETS GROUP: limit these foods, choose lower fat foods with no added sugars

- For a snack or if you're still hungry have one serving of a vegetable and/or a fruit.

- Be sure to always eat in balance: having a protein, grain and fruit or vegetable each meal...

Breakfast

PROTEIN: choose either one serving from the meat/fish/beans/nuts group or one serving from the dairy group*

GRAINS: two servings from the bread, cereal, rice or pasta group*

FRUIT: one serving*

Lunch

PROTEIN : either one serving from the meat/fish/beans/nuts group or one serving from the dairy group (pick from the group you didn't have at breakfast)*

GRAINS : two servings from the bread, cereal, rice or pasta group*

VEGETABLE: one serving*

Dinner

PROTEIN : one serving from both the meat/fish/beans/nuts group and one serving from the dairy group*

GRAINS : two servings from the bread, cereal, rice or pasta group*

VEGETABLE : two servings*

FRUIT : one serving*

- **DRINK six glasses of water a day (eight to ten ounces each)**

- **WAIT twenty minutes after each meal to feel full**

- **EAT VERY SLOWLY. STOP after eating everything on your day's plan. Ask God for help every time.**

*USDA Food Pyramid serving sizes are minimums for most women and older adults. If you are a teenage boy or very active person (thirty or more minutes/day) you may need more servings. Consult with your doctor or dietician/nutritionist to set the right amount to lose between a half and two pounds per week. This plan is not for pregnant or nursing women.

From the book *The Joy of Weight Loss* by Norris Chumley, published by Lantern Books, 2001. Copyright and Trademark 2001 by Norris J. Chumley. All Rights Reserved.

It's a good idea to make several copies of both plans, post them on your refrigerator, carry them with you in your pocketbook or wallet (reduced size, perhaps). Keep your chosen plan at your work place, in your car, everywhere. (Also copy the Joy of Weight Loss Activity Plan onto the other side, while you're at it.)

Now, let's take a little time to explore the six USDA Food Guide Pyramid food groups and find out what a serving size is.

82: Percentage of people who know that a poor diet can increase their risk of cancer.
15: Percentage who have changed their diet to lower that risk.
—Hippocrates Magazine

Eating From All "USDA Food Guide Pyramid" Six Food Groups

The following chart is what the United States Government (the U. S. Department of Agriculture/U.S. Department of Health and Human Services) recommends that an average adult eats every day. It seems like a lot, but when you begin actually doing it, and see what the servings sizes are, it's really not that much—it's just right.

I agree with the USDA Food Guide Pyramid recommendations, and have discovered that if you eat the lower, minimum amount in each food group range, you will slowly lose approximately two pounds per week until you arrive at a reasonable weight for you. (Any more than three pounds per week may not be safe and you should check with your doctor.) Each person is different and everyone's needs vary. How the Joy of Weight Loss Eating plans work are to combine three food groups, protein, grains, and fruits/vegetables all day throughout the day for balanced nutrition. This way, you don't have to keep track of all you need to be healthy and manage your weight. You just eat and naturally get what you need. To know what an "official" serving size is for any particular food, read on. Memorize these serving sizes and, if you have to, use a measuring cup for a couple of weeks to show you exactly how much to have at any given time. Another really good way to gauge serving sizes is to use the palm of your hand. An average human hand's palm is about the equivalent size of two to three ounces of cooked meat. Another way is to imagine a deck of playing cards. That's also about the right equivalent size of two to three ounces of cooked meat.

The idea is to make healthy eating and moderate serving sizes automatic to you. This will happen if you follow the Joy of Weight Loss Eating plans in connection with the USDA Food Guide Pyramid for at least thirty days, like we do together in Chapter 5. In those thirty days, I show you how to gradually begin eating less, meal by meal, week by week. I promise you won't be hungry, you'll feel better, and the weight will come off slowly and surely. All of those results will give you a lot of joy. With God on your side, you'll actually be able to handle all of the joy!

It's not the minutes you take at the table that add to your weight—it's the seconds!

FOOD GUIDE PYRAMID

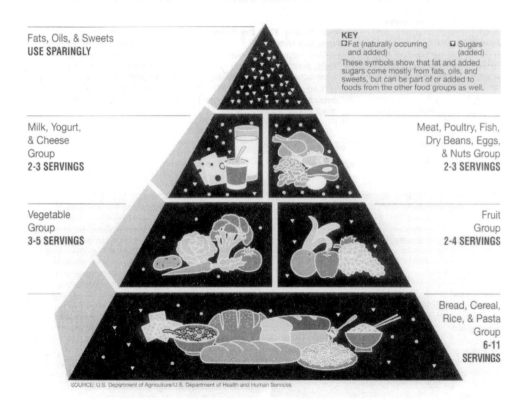

Fats, Oils, & Sweets
USE SPARINGLY

KEY
☐ Fat (naturally occurring and added)   ◘ Sugars (added)
These symbols show that fat and added sugars come mostly from fats, oils, and sweets, but can be part of or added to foods from the other food groups as well.

Milk, Yogurt, & Cheese Group
2-3 SERVINGS

Meat, Poultry, Fish, Dry Beans, Eggs, & Nuts Group
2-3 SERVINGS

Vegetable Group
3-5 SERVINGS

Fruit Group
2-4 SERVINGS

Bread, Cereal, Rice, & Pasta Group
6-11 SERVINGS

SOURCE: U.S. Department of Agriculture/U.S. Department of Health and Human Services

Now, let's go over each group together from the bottom up, and learn the recommended serving sizes. Serving sizes indicated here are those used in the Food Guide Pyramid and based on both suggested and usually consumed portions necessary to achieve adequate intake of nutrients. The serving sizes here differ from those on the Nutrition Facts Label, which reflect portions usually consumed.

Bread, Cereal, Rice and Pasta (Grains)

The foundation of the pyramid is grains. We eat the most of this food group for good reason. Grains are actually starches, which become sugars. We need them to provide energy for our brain, muscles, and central nervous system. Diets consisting of mainly plant-derived grains have been shown to help you avoid chronic diseases like heart disease and cancer. There are various forms of carbohydrates (sugars) from grains, or "carbs." Simple carbohydrates (monosaccharides) are not in grains, but are found in fruits, some vegetables, and honey (eat this kind!). Ordinary table sugar is also a simple sugar, called a disaccharide. Complex carbohydrates (polysaccharides) are pure starches (sugars) found in grains like flour, rice, and pasta and in beans (these are the ones for you!). These also carry plant fiber, which actually isn't digested or absorbed but naturally cleans your system, helps reduce cholesterol, and makes you feel satisfied all day!

Yes, grains contain sugar and we need them. They also carry fiber, which we also need. Caution, however, is required when eating sugars. It is best to eat sugar that also carries fiber and nutrients—like from whole grains, fruits, and vegetables. Sugars from table sugar, alcoholic drinks, candy, desserts, sodas, gum, etc. are "empty calories"— incomplete carbs without fiber or nutrients—and should be limited when you are losing weight. At first, try to eat fewer desserts than you were, and gradually switch to fruits over the course of a few weeks. Make healthy selections for your sweet tooth: foods that contain less concentrated sugars. You will soon get enough sweetness and energy from grains, fruits, and vegetables by eating a small amount at each meal and snack, and you won't crave them. Once you reach your reasonable weight, then it is possible to have some desserts and candy in moderation (like once or twice a week).

GRAIN GROUP SERVING SIZES (Bread, Cereal, Rice, and Pasta)

Gradually lessen your servings and portions until you reach a point where you can have six servings per day during weight loss. A serving is one of the following:

I slice bread *

I ounce ready-to-eat cereal (by weight) *

½ cup cooked cereal, rice or pasta *

I recommend having a grain for each meal and snack; six per day.* This will keep your energy flowing all day long until bedtime, so you'll never feel hungry. You may, of course, vary your servings. For example, if you want to have two grain servings at a meal (a sandwich with two slices of bread, for example), then don't have a grain at the next snack. There's freedom of choice here!

Vegetables

Next on the pyramid that we eat more of than other groups are vegetables. I want you to begin eating more of these than ever before, because they're so good for you. Many scientific studies have confirmed the healthiness of vegetables. That's because they also contain many vitamins, minerals, and fiber that are essential to your good health. But a lot of us don't like the taste of vegetables because we're just not in the habit of eating them—we prefer fatty, salty, or sugary foods because we've been trained that way. To eat more vegetables, try sneaking them into other foods. Add lettuce, tomato, spinach leaves, or pickles to your sandwiches. Throw raw shredded carrots, green peppers, squash, or beans (try chickpeas or kidney beans) into your salads. Have hearty vegetable soups instead of cream or milk-based ones. Try those new delicious combination fruit and vegetable juices (only 100 percent juice, not "drinks")—such as carrot, beet, celery or wheat grass—with fruit juice from apples, oranges, pineapples, or the old delicious stand-by V8 (but not if you have high blood-pressure due to the salt content, or try the

*These recommendations are minimums which are generally appropriate for most women and older adults. If you are a teenage boy or very active man or woman, you may need a greater number of servings. Speak with your doctor or a registered dietician, and experiment week by week to find out exactly the right number of servings for you to safely lose weight at the rate of two to three pounds a week.

newer less sodium version). Don't overcook vegetables. Try light steaming or sautéing them with a touch of garlic and olive oil. You don't need much to satisfy—here's how little a serving is...

VEGETABLE GROUP SERVING SIZES:
Have three servings per day during weight loss.
A serving is one of the following:

I cup raw or leafy vegetables*

½ cup other vegetables—cooked or raw*

¾ cup vegetable juice*

Know that some foods fit into more than one group. Dried beans, peas, and lentils can be considered to be in either the meat and beans group or vegetable group, but in the USDA Food Pyramid they're meat substitutes. Look in the next section on meats where I discuss this further.

Alternate servings of vegetables and fruits with each meal and snack. Therefore, if you have a vegetable for breakfast (like chopped veggies in an omelet, for example), have a fruit for the next snack (like an orange or apple) then a vegetable for lunch. You may certainly mix and match between meals and snacks, but be sure to get at least three servings of vegetables and two servings of fruit in your body during the course of one day. I encourage you to eat lots of vegetables because they're so good for you. If you ever want a second helping, and it's off your food plan, make sure to choose vegetables (or fruit) instead of proteins (which are more heavy laden with calories and fat).

Fruits

I want you to develop a fruit sweet tooth. Replace all of your sweet habits with fruit habits: such as apples, oranges, kiwis, raisins, cherries, grapes, bananas, melons, and berries. Make them your desserts and snacks. Eat an abundance of fruits every day, and you will soon (in a week or less) crave less candy and fewer desserts.

*These recommendations are minimums which are generally appropriate for most women and older adults. If you are a teenage boy or very active man or woman, you may need a greater number of servings. Speak with your doctor or a registered dietician, and experiment week by week to find out exactly the right number of servings for you to safely lose weight at the rate of two to three pounds a week.

Fruit is generally portable, most needs no refrigeration, and it's found anywhere and everywhere. Always pick the freshest, best quality, ripe fruits you can find. Go ahead and spend a little more money to get the best. The money you'll be saving by eating fewer desserts and less candy can be allocated to treat yourself to some fine fruits every day.

Fruits have almost no fat at all compared to proteins, and have far fewer calories than cookies, ice cream, cakes, brownies, candy-bars, and sodas because of their lack of added fat and sugars. Fruits, like vegetables, have lots of vitamins, minerals, and fiber, unlike candy, desserts, and sodas—which have almost no nutritional value whatsoever and lots of concentrated sugar.

When you have a snack, have fruit or a serving of fruit juice (or vegetables) instead of a man-made sweet or baked good. Eating this way is far less harmful than your old sweet habit. If you crave a soda, make yourself a "Joyous Natural Soda" fruit soda:

Joyous Natural Soda
three-quarters of a cup of fruit juice mixed with seltzer or club soda.

FRUIT SERVING SIZES:

Eat two servings per day during weight loss and up to four when managing. Actually, the American Cancer Society recommends nine servings a day of fruits and vegetables.

A USDA Food Pyramid serving is one of the following:

I medium apple, banana, orange, or pear *

½ chopped, cooked or canned fruit *

¾ cup fruit juice *

Alternate fruits and vegetables with each meal and snack. That is, if you have a fruit for breakfast (like bananas on your cereal, for example) have a vegetable for the next snack (how about carrot sticks?) then a fruit for lunch. You may certainly mix and match between meals and snacks, but be sure to get two servings of fruits in your body during the course of one day.

Caution is necessary with fruits if you're diabetic; you don't want too much sugar even if it's from natural fruit sources. As always, check with your physician or registered dietician. You also should be careful not to overdo it on bananas, having no more than one a day.

Proteins

We all need protein to survive, and it can be from meats, poultry, fish, nuts, beans, or dairy products. The USDA Food Guide Pyramid recommends eating a minimum of two servings each from both meat and dairy groups. Again, one serving size is about the size of a deck of playing cards (less than you'd think, right?). If you're a vegetarian you need to make sure to get all of your protein amino acids from combinations of nuts, grains, and beans, or cheese, and enough calcium from green leafy vegetables, supplements, or dairy products. The choice is, of course, up to you. However, I recommend eating as little red and white meat as possible for a lot of reasons. Meat has a lot of saturated fats and may have added hormones and antibiotics. There are also ecological, spiritual, and animal welfare reasons why you may not wish to eat much, if any, meat, but these are beyond the scope of this book.

In the Joy of Weight Loss Eating plans, I recommend having a protein serving in all three meals or three little meals/three little snacks per day, choosing between the meat/nuts/beans group and the dairy group. You should have two servings per day from each group: meat/nuts/beans and dairy. That means, if you had a dairy protein for breakfast, you should have a meat/nuts/beans protein for lunch and then a dairy protein for dinner. For one snack each day, you should have another protein, either in the morning or afternoon. You certainly may mix and match: just get in at least two meat/nut/bean and two dairy group servings in you over the course of a day. Have your protein however you like, in whatever foods you like. Just eat a small amount. Simple.

> *To be without some of the things you want is an indispensable part of happiness.*
>
> —Bertrand Russell

*These recommendations are minimums which are generally appropriate for most women and older adults. If you are a teenage boy or very active man or woman, you may need a greater number of servings. Speak with your doctor or a registered dietician, and experiment week by week to find out exactly the right number of servings for you to safely lose weight at the rate of two to three pounds a week.

Meat and Beans Group
(meat, poultry, fish, dried beans, eggs, and nuts)

Be careful of this group: only eat a little! Protein (amino acids and nitrogen) is crucial to our survival because it nourishes muscles, skin, tissues, and virtually all parts of our bodies. However, protein from animals carries a lot of saturated fat, the kind that raises your cholesterol levels which can make you saturated with fat! You do need protein and some fat, but most of us get way too much. If you look at certain ethnic populations, such as Asians, many who eat little or no meat and, if they do, use it only for flavoring, they have fewer weight problems. We should learn from them.

The USDA recommends two to three servings of meat, poultry, fish, eggs, nuts, or beans. Many experts think even this is too much. But a serving is actually only two to three ounces cooked. I honestly recommend you eat little or no red meat, and stick with poultry, fish, nuts, and beans. You'll be healthier in the long run. If you must have red meat because you crave it, have it only once or twice a week at the most. Choose lean cuts, of the highest quality you can get. (I did not have any red meat for ten years and only recently decided to have a little in my life. I've always been healthier from eating less meat, and my cholesterol levels show it.) You may wish to have at least two servings of fish or shellfish per week, and more if possible. You should limit egg yolks to two a week because they have a lot of cholesterol. Nuts contain no saturated fat, which is good, but they are far more fatty for the amount of protein you get from them. I would highly recommend eating beans! Try chickpeas, white beans, pinto, black-eyed peas, soybeans, tofu: Experiment! Keep an open mind. If you get gas from beans, try gradually adding them to your diet, or experiment with different methods of cooking them.

MEAT AND BEANS GROUP SERVING SIZE: (meat, poultry, fish, nuts, and beans)

Have two servings per day during weight loss. A serving is one of the following:

Two to three ounces cooked, lean meat, poultry or fish (the size of a deck of playing cards)*

½ cup of cooked dry beans or ½ cup of tofu counts as 1 ounce of lean meat*

2½-ounce soyburger or 1 egg counts as 1 ounce of lean meat*

Two tablespoons of peanut butter or ⅓ cup of nuts counts as 1 ounce of meat*

*These recommendations are minimums which are generally appropriate for most women and older adults. If you are a teenage boy or very active man or woman, you may need a greater number of servings. Speak with your doctor or a registered dietician, and experiment week by week to find out exactly the right number of servings for you to safely lose weight at the rate of two to three pounds a week.

Know that some foods fit into more than one group. Dried beans, peas, and lentils can be counted as servings in either the meat and beans group or vegetable group. These "cross over" foods can be counted as servings from either one or the other group, but not both. As a vegetable, half a cup of cooked, dry beans counts as one serving. As a meat substitute, one cup of cooked, dry beans counts as one serving (two ounces of meat).

Dairy Group

A lot of people avoid dairy products, because they are worried about the fat content or have lactose intolerace, and rightfully so. Dairy products do contain fat, and as with meats it's the saturated type because it's animal in origin. However, milk products also contain calcium, the bony-white mineral that our bones need to stay hard. As we get older we face the risk of osteoporosis—brittle bone disease—which can be avoided if you have your calcium every day. You can get it from other sources: green vegetables like spinach, collards, or kale; from various beans; or from edible bony fish such as salmon or sardines. You can also get calcium-enriched soy milk, which also has essential vitamins like B$_{12}$ and D. However, calcium may be harder to get from these foods because they carry less calcium and the body may not absorb them as well. So have some dairy products every day, and know that you don't need a lot, only two servings (three if you're under twenty-four, or are pregnant or nursing. But, just to remind you, never attempt a weight loss program when you're expecting or you've just given birth). If you're worried about fat, have low-fat or fat-free (skim) milk, yogurt, or white low-fat cheese.

Some of us (like me) are on the other side of the fence with dairy products. We love them too much! Milk, cheese, and ice cream are all "trigger" foods for me, and for a lot of people I know and work with. I believe that it was my nightly ice cream habit that really caused me to be obese. Dairy products need to be eaten sparingly for those of us who are crazy for them, because large amounts on a regular basis add a lot of fat to your body. Two servings a day are enough. Certainly, if you're a cheese or ice cream junkie, it would pay for you to ask God to help you avoid them entirely. When I was losing my weight, I was able to enjoy God's grace and not crave or eat ice cream for a very long time. Even now, I only have it perhaps once or twice a month, and thankfully my compulsion for it has been lifted for over a decade.

(Milk, yogurt, and cheese—This includes lactose-free and lactose-reduced milk products. One cup of soy-based beverage with added calcium is an option for those who prefer a non-dairy source of calcium.)

Have two servings per day during weight loss (up to three when managing). A serving is one of the following. Choose fat-free or reduced-fat dairy products most often.

1 cup milk or yogurt*

1 ½ ounces natural cheese*

2 ounces processed cheese*

Try, if possible, to choose dairy foods that are free of hormones and pesticides, such as organics or milk from certified hormone-free cows.

About Lactose Intolerance

Some folks do not tolerate milk and dairy products well, and experience nausea, cramps, bloating, gas, and diarrhea about one-half hour to two hours after eating or drinking food containing lactose (the significant sugar in milk). This is due to lack of an ability to digest the lactose, due to a shortage of the enzyme lactase, produced by cells that line the small intestine. If you are "lactose intolerant" you probably know it already, but if you frequently have these symptoms ask your doctor. There are several simple tests which can help you find out.

According to the National Digestive Diseases Information Clearing House, between thirty to fifty million people have this problem, which is actually quite manageable if you know what to eat. As many as seventy percent of all African-Americans and Native Americans, and ninety percent of Asian-Americans are lactose intolerant. These folks may wish to try calcium-enriched soy milk. The problem is least common among persons of northern European descent. In addition, the University of California Wellness letter makes this recommendation:

---

*These recommendations are minimums which are generally appropriate for most women and older adults. If you are a teenage boy or very active man or woman, you may need a greater number of servings. Speak with your doctor or a registered dietician, and experiment week-by-week to find out exactly the right number of servings for you to safely lose weight at the rate of two to three pounds a week.

Young children with lactase deficiency should not eat any foods containing lactose. Most older children and adults need not avoid lactose completely, but individuals differ in the amounts of lactose they can handle. For example, one person may suffer symptoms after drinking a small glass of milk, while another can drink one glass but not two. Others may be able to manage ice cream and aged cheeses, such as cheddar and Swiss but not other dairy products. Dietary control of lactose intolerance depends on each person's learning through trial and error how much lactose he or she can handle.

For those who react to very small amounts of lactose or have trouble limiting their intake of foods that contain lactose, lactase enzymes are available without a prescription. One form is a liquid for use with milk. A few drops are added to a quart of milk, and after twenty-four hours in the refrigerator, the lactose content is reduced by seventy percent. The process works faster if the milk is heated first, and adding a double amount of lactase liquid produces milk that is ninety percent lactose free. A more recent development is a chewable lactase enzyme tablet that helps people digest solid foods that contain lactose. Three to six tablets are taken just before a meal or snack.

Lactose-reduced milk and other products are available at many supermarkets. The milk contains all of the nutrients found in regular milk and remains fresh for about the same length of time or longer if it is super-pasteurized.

Even older women at risk for osteoporosis and growing children who must avoid milk and foods made with milk can meet most of their special dietary needs by eating greens, fish, and other calcium-rich foods that are free of lactose. A carefully chosen diet (with calcium supplements if the doctor or dietitian recommends them) is the key to reducing symptoms and protecting future health.

Drinks

This is a really easy category. The simple answer is to drink a lot! A lot of water! You should have at least six large glasses (eight to ten ounces) per day. This could be tap water, bottled, "designer," carbonated, flavored, any kind you like—but just make sure it's unsweetened and unsalted. If it's tap water you're drinking, let it run for two minutes before drinking to lower the possibility of lead contamination. Avoid club soda, because of the added salt, and have seltzer instead. I know, however, seltzer is sometimes hard to find outside of big cities. Limit or avoid spritzer or "light" drinks because of the added sugar or artificial sweeteners.

Please **do not drink any diet drinks of any kind**. They all have chemicals and artificial sweeteners that have not been on this Earth long enough for us to know if they're safe. Lots and lots of people have severe medical reactions to them. If you don't believe me, look at the warnings on the labels. That should be enough to scare you away! A friend of mine once said: "If cancer had a flavor, it'd taste like diet soda!" Actually, science isn't sure whether diet drinks cause cancer or any adverse health problems, and a recent study disproved the decades old impression that they did. But why take a chance? Drink the tried and true drinks—like water, fruit and vegetable juices, tea and coffee in moderate amounts. If you crave sodas, make fruit sodas (three-quarters of a cup of juice and sparkling water mixed) and count them as a fruit serving.

Be careful of bottled fruit "drinks," fruit sodas, or iced-tea drinks—they usually contain a lot of sugar and there is more than one serving in a bottle. If you must have these drinks, count them as two or more carbohydrate (grain) servings. While I believe it is better to have real fruit juice, you should be careful of fruit juice, too! It's easy to have too much. Most "individual bottles" have two or three servings packed in them and often have added sugars. Also beware of fruit "drinks"—these contain mostly water, sugar, and just a small amount of juice. Wasted calories, again! Read the labels.

Coffee and teas are fine. I love them, too. But again, the middle, moderate path is for you. That means have a maximum of only two cups of coffee or caffeinated tea a day—because you don't want too much caffeine. A tablespoon of non-fat or low-fat milk is OK, if you like. Avoid sugar or artificial sweeteners when you're losing weight. Herbal teas are sublime, and green tea is divine! (Remember though, green tea is often caffeinated.) According to some authorities, one to two cups of green tea per day can cut down the risks of getting cancer and heart-disease.

As for alcoholic beverages, it is best to avoid them all together when losing weight. This is because they're metabolized as sugar but carry no additional nutrients. They're wasted calories, again. Moreover, the effects of alcohol sometimes leave you throwing caution and reason to the wind. It's a lot easier to overeat when you're tipsy!

If you must, alcoholic beverages are OK to have and count as a carbohydrate (grain) during the weight management phase of your life. However, I recommend having them only in moderation, as with everything. Moderation might mean a limit of two servings a week, or, at the most, one glass of beer or wine per day. (The French have done this for generations, and enjoy good health!)

Recreational Drugs and Medications

There are several habits that I should mention that will truly cause your weight problem to be worse. Using recreational drugs is a particularly bad habit, especially the use of marijuana. You may've heard of "the munchies." It's when you've had pot, and a little while later your blood sugar plummets and you crave food, particularly sweets. Gotta have them and gotta have a lot, immediately. People I've worked with who use marijuana frequently struggle with weight problems, not to mention depression and apathy. Painkillers, tranquilizers, and "downers" can also trigger out-of-control eating. Some prescription drugs can cause weight gain. If you're regularly taking any medication or recreational drug, be aware that it may have weight side-effects. This could be a part of your problem. It is much better to get your tranquility and joy from living, being active, having friends, and being with God. The only side-effects are positive!

Snacks

You must have snacks! They are essential if you are to feel full and nourished with enough energy and vigor to keep you going throughout the day. I want you to eat between meals, just a little, two to three hours after a meal. However, I want you to have healthy snacks, not manufactured "snack foods," because they're chock full of fat, salt, and sugar (it's sometimes amazing to me they even call them "foods" because they often have little nutritional value). You can have either a fruit or vegetable and a grain, three times a day, depending on which Joy of Weight Loss Eating plan you've chosen for the day, and what you have or haven't had during the rest of the day. If you haven't had enough fruit (two servings) you should have them at snack time; if you haven't had enough vegetables (three servings) snack time is catch-up time. It is the same deal with protein.

My favorite snack is a sourdough pretzel and an apple. Or you could have crackers and grapes, a piece of bread with pure-fruit spread on it (unsweetened, if possible), cut-up carrot-sticks, or green peppers and a little left-over pasta or rice. Maybe there's half a turkey sandwich in the fridge you could have, or a left-over piece of quiche. Or you could stop at a bagel place and have half a bagel with a little vegetable cream cheese on it. Bagels are great, but their size varies widely in a range of one to six ounces. The big ones are actually two servings or as much as three servings of grains.

Have your snack with a big glass of water, for fullness. For one snack a day, add a little protein, either from the meat and nut or the dairy groups, if you're on the Three Meals/Three Snacks Plan. I recommend having the protein either in the morning or afternoon (it's your choice) whenever you need a long-lasting energy boost. You could have cheese and crackers, or sliced baked tofu on a piece of bread, or popcorn and peanuts. I recommend that you do not have the protein just before bed for reasons of digestion (or indigestion!). Finish eating at least two hours before retiring.

Eating snacks is wise because doing so will keep your blood-sugar and proteins at the right levels all day long. Also, you won't feel that intense desire to overeat late in the day.

About Fats and Sweets

It's OK! You are allowed some "goodies." You gave up dieting forever, remember? God has liberated you by your consistent requests for help, remember? You may occasionally have your pizza, your cheese sandwiches, hamburgers, French fries, and even ice cream. Don't worry, you will not have to give them up entirely. What you do need to do, however, is be aware which foods have a lot of fat, salt, and sugar and just not have a lot of them. Keep the serving sizes honest; be aware of how much you're eating of these foods—like you are with everything else. That's all. Keep following the Joy of Weight Loss Eating plans and just fit them into it. This means that you'll only have one of these things at a time. Have a slice of pizza with meat or veggies on top for lunch. But only have one slice. Eat it slowly and savor each little bite. Have a hamburger and French fries for dinner (even from a fast food joint), and add lettuce and tomato and pickles between the bun. What's different, though, is that, if you follow my plan, you won't want to choose the giant size portion. You should keep each meat serving the size of a deck of playing cards, eat really slowly, and not have a chocolate shake with it! (Have plain carbonated water, or unsweetened iced tea.)

Keep an eye out for too much fat and sugar carbohydrates, by reading the labels on sides of boxes and wrappers. Take time to stop, look, and read before you eat too much of something that may not be so good for you. It's will also be fruitful time well-spent to read a book or two on nutrition (there are some ever-updated suggestions on my website, www.NorrisChumley.com or www.JoyOfWeightLoss.com).

Just as you shouldn't overdose on the bad stuff, you shouldn't go overboard and zealously eliminate all fat and sugar from your life. Eating no-fat, chemically treated diet food, or only fruit and vegetables all of a sudden is a recipe for disaster and failure. Again, the idea is to be simple, moderate, reasonable, and kind to your body and your psyche. Take the middle road—not too much and not too little—and you will manage your weight for the long-term. You will also joyfully enrich your life.

Here are some easy ways to reduce fats in your life:

- trim away fats from meats before or after cooking

- cook foods in a non-stick pan, use water to steam, or have just one teaspoon of oil wiped onto the pan with a paper towel. (Use non-saturated vegetable oils such as olive, canola, corn, or peanut instead of lard, palm, or cottonseed oils.)

- Use vegetable, chicken, or fish bouillon to cook with instead of creamy sauces.

- Use half or one-quarter the amount of butter you would ordinarily use. I would not use margarine (it contains hydrogenated, "trans-fatty" acids that some authorities have suggested may be harmful for your long-term health).

Here are some easy ways to reduce sugars in your life:

- Have yogurt, sorbet, or sherbet (if you must) instead of ice cream.

- To indulge your sweet tooth, have one piece of something: a hard candy, or cube of chocolate, or graham crackers, gingersnaps, or animal cookies. Better yet, eat a piece of fruit.

- Have flavored water (unsweetened) instead of sodas. Or one glass of iced tea, with a squeeze of fruit and one teaspoon of sugar.

There are, however, certain food cravings that we cannot control. Everyone has them, and it's not fun or joyful to deal with them. Some of us are particularly vulnerable to becoming addicted to these "trigger" or "binge" foods.

"Trigger" Foods

Is there one kind of food or food group that controls you—a food that you absolutely have to have all of the time, that you eat way too much of but can't stop indulging in? For some people it's chips, others ice cream, sodas, nuts, desserts, or baked-goods. One thing for sure, however, triggers are rarely foods that are healthy for you in large quantities. I don't know a single person who's addicted to vegetables, do you?!

If you're compulsive with any food (habitually driven, addicted, and must urgently have it all the time) then you have a serious problem that you need to face head-on. It could be the cause of your weight problems. It may be subtle and you may not even be aware of it. An example is a soda habit—drinking just one large soda every day can add three to five pounds to your body per month. (Did you know that there are ten teaspoons of sugar in a regular size soda? Shocking, right?) Or it might be a fat/sugar/salt food habit, where you are always eating high-fat, salty, or high-sugar foods for every meal (deep-fat fried foods, meats, milk-shakes, desserts, pastries, cream, mayonnaise, or buttery things). These will definitely cause you to be overweight.

The compulsive "trigger" food problem may be obvious. You may be like I used to be with ice cream. My need to have a pint or even half a gallon to get to sleep meant I was taking in the equivalent of all of the calories and fats that a normal weight person would have in one or even two days of eating. I knew this was a serious problem, but I couldn't control it; instead, it controlled me. After years of compulsive struggling, watching my weight go up and my quality of life go down, I could only do one thing. Ask God for help.

I said a prayer to God, surrendering everything in order to be freed of this horrible compulsion. I was serious. I had to give up, because nothing else I had tried worked. I was desperate. Because of my surrender, I was liberated. Not only was the compulsion lifted, I wasn't even attracted to my trigger food anymore. I no longer needed it. The extreme blessing I received was to actually be neutral about ice cream. No, I haven't sworn off it forever; that would be extreme and unrealistic. I've now got the spiritual power to be realistic and reasonable, and not addicted anymore because of God's gift to me. I have ice cream once in a while, and it's no big deal. I can easily sleep without it, because I fill my mind with sweet thoughts of God and my appreciation of the blessings I've received over and over again. That is the Joy of Weight Loss for me. Food addictions are not easy problems to deal with. Unlike addictions to other substances such as alcohol, cigarettes, and drugs, we cannot simply stop eating food. We have to eat. Unlike an alcoholic or drug addict who must completely end their consumption of their trigger substances, we must learn to continue eating in a responsible, controlled manner. That's why many of us say recovering from compulsive overeating is the most difficult problem to overcome. That's why few are able to do it, and why miracles are often necessary from the hand of God.

You can easily be rid of your "trigger" foods, too. You can feel the honest joy of relief and never have to be compulsive over them again. You need to start by realizing and admitting their power over you. You need to feel the pain and side-effects associated with constantly eating the trigger food or foods, tied into the temporary pleasure. Allow yourself to tap into the deep emotions that may be linked to eating these foods. You're doing it for a reason, after all. You're doing it not only out of habit, but because these trigger foods give you comfort on some level. Do you have any childhood memories associated with these foods? (Ice cream, as we've seen, was for me emotionally linked to times when I felt my mother's love.) Do you have any feelings of being cared for when you eat your trigger foods? Is fried chicken a symbol of emotional safety and happiness for you? Are French fries tokens of affection? Is cake a reminder of parties and happy moments? Make the mental association, see the link, and find the cause of your addiction. Then surrender that addiction to God, in a solemn desire to find happiness, comfort, safety, pleasure, and *joy* in ways that aren't going to make you or keep you fat and in bondage to your compulsions.

Slips, Mistakes, Binges, and Failures

There are no such things as mistakes on this plan. You cannot screw up. It's impossible! If you are honestly doing your best to stay with the plan, giving your problems to God, and being moderately active every day, over time everything will be just fine. Even if you temporarily go off the plan once in a while, it's OK, because you can make up for it the next meal. Here's how:

- If you eat too much of one thing, eat less of it next time.

- If you binge, then skip the next meal or have only half servings.

- If you find yourself craving more food at certain times, make sure you're having enough at meals and at snack time. Or reallocate servings from one meal or snack to the time that you need them.

- If you miss a day of being active, pick it up the next and keep "getting started." Don't let a one- or two-day slip be the end of your active life.

The Joy of Weight Loss is not about being perfect. That's impossible. It's about enjoying eating from all food groups in moderation, throughout the day, in your own time and individual caring way. *It's about the whole picture, the sum of a month's worth of eating* in a healthy, moderate way. Rethink your eating habits toward a monthly average, not what you've eaten at one meal or in a day. That way, the pressure is off, you can self-adjust, and follow God's subtle directions over time. Just do your best, follow your good intentions, relax and allow yourself to make some mistakes, and ask God to show you what to do to correct them, forgive them, and learn from them. This way, when you make a mistake again, you won't punish yourself so much.

Read the labels

Although the U.S. government has spent a lot of time, energy, and money trying to standardize and improve food product labeling, the "Nutrition Facts" labels are still somewhat confusing. Serving sizes on these labels are still not standard, and often "standard" is just what the manufacturer chooses as a "typical" size or an amount "usually consumed." Manufacturers quote their serving sizes notoriously small, and make multiple servings per container so you'll think the product is low-calorie or low-fat—which it often isn't. If only the serving sizes would correlate with the USDA Food Guide Pyramid, then it'd all be easier. But they mostly don't, and, because of this confusion and because I do not want you to obsess about calories, fat, vitamins or minerals, I suggest you only read the labels in a "moderate" kind of way. Be educated about what you're eating but don't worry about tracking everything. Stick with your Joy of Weight Loss Eating Plan and USDA Food Guide Pyramid recommendations above for food groups and serving sizes.

This is how you find some "moderate" value in a label:

- Check the size of the item. How many ounces is it or what's its weight? When you have found that out, convert the measurement to your own serving size guidelines. (Pay no attention to the label's serving size and number of servings; they don't mean much.) You're looking for cups: half, three-quarters, one cup. If you don't actually have a measuring cup with you, just make an estimation.

- Look at the calories and the calories from fat. Although these figures relate to the manufacturer's non-standardized serving sizes, you can still see if the product has high calories or fat. The most useful thing you can do is approximate the percentage of fat in the product as related to the calories. If it's a 100-calorie item, and the calories from fat is fifty, then it's fifty percent fat. That means the item is not one you want to eat a lot of.

- Briefly glance at the "below-the-line" figures, looking immediately to the right in the "% daily value" column. What does this product have the most of? Is it mainly fat, protein, or carbohydrates? Does it have a high salt (sodium) percentage? How are the cholesterol levels, saturated fat, fiber, sugar, minerals?

Then, at the bottom, look at the vitamins and minerals. What percentage of your "Daily Values" does this product provide? (Again, "Daily Values" are somewhat confusing, too. They're based on what the government establishes as minimums. But many health professionals think they're too low or too high. Just eat well, from all six USDA Food Pyramid food groups, take a daily vitamin, and you'll be fine. Simplicity is best!)

- Obviously, not every food has a Nutrition Facts label. It would be a good idea to get a nutrition book, or calorie and fat counter, as a healthy addition to your food education. Just as long as you don't go overboard or worry about it.

Vitamins?

As I mentioned above, I recommend taking a daily multi-vitamin, just to make sure you're getting the basics covered. Sure, obviously if you eat a balanced healthful diet of everything recommended you'll get what you need in the way of nutrients, vitamins, and minerals, but it can't hurt to be sure. Take your ordinary, over-the-counter drugstore vitamin tablet in the morning just after breakfast, and preferably not on a full stomach.

There are some "experts" out there who recommend loading up on specific vitamins or taking large doses of minerals or suppliments of various kinds, with a myriad of claims. But I think common sense should rule, and you shouldn't overdo it. I believe in moderation in every way, including vitamins. Don't take a chance: some vitamins or minerals in large quantities can make you sick, cause health problems over time, or even be fatal in rare cases.

If you think you do need more than a multi-vitamin, as always, ask your personal physician or registered dietician.

Now What?

I have included a list of food ideas for you to choose from at the back of the book, which illustrate both Joy Of Weight Loss food plans, so you can have an idea of what and how much you may want to eat each day.

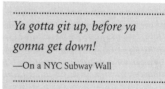

Ya gotta git up, before ya gonna get down!
—On a NYC Subway Wall

THE JOY OF BEING ACTIVE

We all know that we have to move. We have to use our bodies, exercise them, stretch and tone our muscles, energize the nerves, keep the blood flowing and the heart pumping. If we don't we'll feel stiff and achy, gain weight, and eventually have a much higher chance of developing serious or fatal illnesses at an unfairly young age. There's just no other way around it—use it or lose it!

All people should exercise, but for the right reasons: to improve the cardiovascular system; to improve the strength, endurance, and flexibility of the muscular system; and to effect positive changes on other body systems such as the skeletal, digestive, and immune systems, and for other manifestations of improved health such as lower serum lipids and lower blood pressure.

—National Academy of Sciences

So, if we have to exercise, we might as well enjoy it. We might as well make moving and being active a source of joy and happiness.

Again, the key is to surrender. Give up your old beliefs that exercise is torture. While you're at it, forget calling it exercise ever again! Forget the concept of "pain is gain." Pain is pain and it's a signal that something's wrong! Let go of the excuse: "There's never enough time." We are now going to forever change the way you think about using your body. Actually, I'd like you to *only think of moving as being something that you enjoy*—a luxurious yet necessary gift that you want to give yourself every day.

Being active on a daily basis gives you:

- More energy
- A clear mind
- Good feelings, elevated moods
- Decreased appetite
- A slower aging process
- A way to help prevent diseases
- Deeper, more restful sleep
- Skin quality: firmness, fewer wrinkles, elasticity, color
- Less stiffness, muscle and bone aches, tension
- Accelerated weight loss
- Lifetime weight management

Movement Myths

The hardest part is just to get started every day and to find time to do it. It's just not true that you have to do intense or vigorous exercise to see some results. Nor do you have to spend hours a day at the gym, or be "perfectly in shape" in order to be healthy and maintain a reasonable weight.

Once you overcome the inertia of starting, once you're engaged in activity, joy arrives and you experience great pleasure. It's the extra endorphins (the "happy" chemicals) in your brain getting secreted from using your muscles. Being active makes

For people who exercise rarely or not at all, short but frequent bouts of aerobic exertion can improve fitness somewhat. In one study, for example, sedentary subjects were able to increase their aerobic capacity by about fifteen percent in three months by running in place for just ten minutes a day.

—University of California Wellness Letter

you feel high! Athletes call it the "second wind." But you don't have to be an athlete to get it. As a matter of fact, you don't even have to move much—even just walking every day will get the body moving and the emotions freed-up, giving you a lot of joy. You can also do something a little more vigorous, but not too hard—like playing a simple game, such as tossing a ball with a friend, or a little tennis or squash, dancing around the house, or an easy swim. You don't need to be good at sports or even physically coordinated. Often, just getting outside and into nature will bring you a terrific feeling of joy, in addition to airing your lungs, opening your eyes, and clearing the mind. The point is just to be "moderately" active on a consistent, daily basis, and enjoy being healthy and active.

> *Those who do not find time for exercise will have to find time for illness.*
> —Edward Stanley

1. *The trick is to get addicted to daily activity.* "Exercising" for the majority of people isn't fun, and we just won't do it long-term. The concept of "exercise" needs to be reframed into "enjoyable activity." If you dedicate yourself to being active, having fun, and feeling good, then you will want to move every day, for a lifetime. *Don't do any activity that you do not enjoy! But do something every day that you do!*

2. Start slowly, but make a commitment to be active every day and to enjoy it. No matter what happens, promise God and yourself that you will move today and that you'll do everything possible to find joy in your physical activities.

3. Get started every morning. Before you have breakfast, or just after, schedule time to be active by fitting it into your existing schedule. Start with just ten minutes, and then build up and increase your joyful activity time each week. (Follow the Joy of Weight Loss Daily Companion for help. Keep a log, too, and praise yourself every day for doing it.) If you can't fit activity into your morning schedule, then do it during your lunch break, or after work. Just do it!

The Joy of Weight Loss Activity Plan

You know by now that in order to really lose weight, and maintain it once you've done it, you need to be active every day. The best way to do that is to **surrender your old habits and preconceptions to God and integrate daily physical activity into your lifestyle.** *I want you to love moving so much that you cannot live without it. Because that's the truth—you can't!*

Slowly, over one to two months, build up to:

- **A minimum of thirty minutes daily of moderate activity: walking, dancing, swimming, racquet sports, golf, housework, fishing, bicycling, canoeing, home improvement, etc. You can do more vigorous activities—such as aerobics, cardiovascular conditioning, running or jogging, water or snow skiing, sledding, gardening, or competitive sports, etc.—if you wish.**

- **Choose whatever you like. Vary activities day by day (as I do), making them a part of your lifestyle.** *Just be active every day.*

If you're at the point where you're being active every day, but not up to thirty minutes, or if you've worked up to the recommended length of time, but just not every day, I want to encourage you to break through your barriers.

- **Make activity a high priority for reasons of health: to get more energy, to slow down aging, maintain stable weight, live longer, and to feel better. Other than family or God, there's probably nothing more important. Without your health, you have nothing.**

- **Improve your emotions, handle stress, look better through daily activity.**

There are many ways to do it. Open up, get creative, and ask God to help you get into it every day. While it's important to be active on a daily basis, again, moderation is essential. *Keep your active play time to no more than one hour per day.* It's not a good idea to overdo it; you won't benefit from it and you may hurt yourself. Also, if you ever feel dizzy, in pain, winded, or gasping for breath, slow down or stop what you're doing. If you're exerting yourself beyond the point where you cannot speak or carry on a conversation, you're pushing yourself too much.

Before beginning a daily activity program, it's vitally important that you get your physician's approval and assurance that what you propose for yourself is going to be safe and healthy.

ALWAYS BEGIN YOUR DAILY ACTIVITY WITH A WARMUP AND STRETCH!

Before you begin, take five minutes to stretch both to warm up and avoid injury.

Calves: stand an arm's length away from a wall, then lean with both forearms on the wall bent at the elbows, stretching one leg directly behind you (one at a time!) as far as you can. Resist the urge to bounce; it's not good for your muscles.

Thighs: now stand straight against the wall, reach one arm behind your leg and grab your ankle from behind. Pull your foot toward your butt, gently, as far as is comfortable. Feel the thigh stretch. Hold it for thirty seconds per leg.

Arms and Back: while still standing, reach both arms toward the ceiling. Hold for thirty seconds. Now do one arm at a time, stretching the arms and back, reaching high to the ceiling (but don't bounce). Do this five times on each arm.

Neck: turn your head and look all the way to the right, then to the left five times each. Now look up to the ceiling and then down to the ground for five times.

Shoulders: rotate both your shoulders toward the front five times, and then toward the back another five times.

Fingers: hold your arms out straight in front of you and flex the fingers of both hands in and out ten times.

Hamstrings (the back leg muscles): sit on the floor with your legs and feet out in front of you. Now slowly reach your arms toward your toes. Only go as far as is comfortable, and just a tiny bit more.

BE SURE TO ALWAYS BREATHE DEEPLY WHILE STRETCHING AND DURING ACTIVITY.

Post this plan everywhere. Make copies, and add them to the back of the Joy of Weight Loss Eating Plan. Post them at home, carry them with you, put them in your car and desk. And do it!

> Ten minutes of exercise performed four days per week for six weeks may be more important than six weeks of thirty-minute sessions that vary between one to five times per week because the person is developing a consistent pattern of exercise.

Building Activity Into Your Life

Observe your dog: if he's fat, you're not getting enough exercise!

You don't need to do your daily activity all at once. You may split it into ten or twenty minute bursts. Vary your activities and the levels of intensity.

There are ways to be active without spending hours at the gym or on exercise machines half the day. Often, just changing your overall mindset to an "active" lifestyle and being physical wherever and whenever possible, instead of being passive and physically minimal, works wonders. Here are some ideas:

AT HOME:
- Walk to the post office, mall, or grocery store, then home (or just one way, and take a bus or taxi home). Walk to pick-up the kids from school and walk home with them.

- Paint a room that needs it.

- Plant and maintain a garden and weed it every day.

- Carry books around with you, as weights, and lift them.

- Vacuum, mop, or scrub more often. Be more thorough, slow, and deliberate, like your grandmother was. Chop wood, dig ditches, build stuff like your grandfather did.

- Wash some clothes by hand, like your great grandmother!

- Dance to CD's, tapes, the radio, or TV.

- Go to a mall and walk the perimeter, before you shop.

- Plan and play more physical games with the family—tossing balls, soccer (play don't just always watch), tennis, badminton, volleyball, softball, swimming, water or snow skiing, rowing or paddle boating, basketball, lacrosse, squash, racquetball, etc.

- Go to a park and take a power walk. Bring the family or friends.

On the National Weight Control Registry study of 773 successful weight loss maintainers, many engaged in walking the equivalent of twenty-eight miles per week!

AT THE OFFICE:

- Suggest a "walking meeting" to your colleagues. Instead of sitting around the board room table, walk and talk your plans and decisions.

- Instead of asking others to run your errands, run them yourself.

- Enroll in a corporate activity program. Many corporations and companies provide one at little or no cost—as a benefit perk—and allow you time in the day to use it.

- Walk up stairs and down, instead of using elevators or escalators all the time.

- Park your car a few blocks away or at the edge of the parking lot or on the top floor of the garage and walk the extra distance.

- Stand on the bus or commuter train instead of sitting. (Standing uses more muscles and burns a few more calories.)

- Join or organize an office "fun league," and play some easy, but fun sport once or twice a week together. You can play volleyball, softball, soccer, basketball, or have dancing groups—swing, Latin, ballroom, whatever! Just emphasize health and fun, not competition or proving one's athletic prowess.

- Or, have a company power walk (or just with a few friends) for half an hour before work every morning or several times a week. Make commitments to each other to stick with it and to motivate each other, rain or shine, all the time.

I strongly recommend enrolling in a recreation class. I've done this for a decade and absolutely love modern, ballroom, and Latin dance classes, water aerobics, racquetball and squash classes. I've made a lot of friends, and have had many, many hours of total pleasure. Many people I've helped have done this with good results as well.

Try some newer recreational activities, like:

- Weightlifting, but not with heavy weights. Many repetitions with light weights can help tone you up. Try a body sculpting class or work with a personal coach.

- Rebounding—mini-trampoline

- Spinning—intense bicycling to music

- Tai Chi/boxing—combining ancient Asian movement arts with boxing

- Water dancing—ballet, jazz, or modern dance underwater

- Rock climbing—machines or walls

- Fitness "camps"—basic training; variety of exercises to music

- Latin dancing

- Hip hop/club dancing

- Ballroom or square dancing

- Body sculpting

- Yoga

- Stair-climbing

- The Pilates Method—a new form of stretching and toning

The way to get into it every day is to get into a routine. Make the effort to overcome your plateaus, blocks, fears, lethargy, busy-ness, and just make it a priority. Allow one to two months of effort, by being moderately, easily active on a daily basis, and then you'll be hooked.

If I can do it, you can. I went from being a 400-pound totally sedentary person, to a completely fit and healthy, happy, active person. I wouldn't miss a day for anything. You don't need to either.

Here are some ways to get you going and keep you motivated, to the point of healthy addiction.

> *An early morning walk is a blessing for the whole day.*
> —Henry David Thoreau

Essential: Commit to moving each and every day for yourself and for God. Although you promise yourself on a daily basis, make sure to keep it up for at least one month. Get that pleasurable high and overall feeling of fitness.

Best: Be active with a trainer or with a friend. Make a pact to be active and have fun together at least once a week. You motivate each other, talk while you're moving, it goes quickly, and it's more enjoyable.

> *How can God direct our steps if we're not taking any?*
> —Sarah Leah Grafstein

Better: Play and have fun with several friends, and/or with co-workers twice a week, so that you have someone to go with every time. It's a joy for everyone involved.

Great: Take group activity classes at a school, university, YMCA, hospital or community recreation center. Sign up for at least two times a week, hopefully more, and pre-pay for several months (and possibly get a discount) if you can. Start with a really easy class, like "stretch and movement," "beginner's yoga," "water ballet," or "ballroom dancing." (A common mistake is to take a hard class and get discouraged.) Classes are cheap, fun, you'll meet friends, and receive a lot of attention and motivation. One caveat: you need to get there every time—that's the challenge. Again, commitment to health, fitness, and pleasure will do it.

Even Greater: Work with a personal consultant or trainer, twice or three times per week. Private ones can be expensive but are worth it if it's in your budget. Try your local school, university, YMCA, or community recreation center—there you may find inexpensive, committed helpers. (Hint: some colleges or universities have recreational education students who need practice—they sometimes work for college credit or very little money.)

You Are Naturally A Part of Nature

When you go outside for a walk, let yourself feel the joy of being in nature. Open your eyes and your heart and soul to new living things. See the living colors of the green grass, the leaves on trees and plants, the radiant flowers, the blue sky and white clouds. Breathe deep the fresh air. Let the energy of the sun shine down on your skin and into your eyes for a few moments. Hear the birds singing and the bugs buzzing. Feel the fresh kiss of a living lawn or the mud of all life between your fingers. Sip water from a flowing river or let the ocean waves caress your toes one after another. Smell the new mown hay in the country, the pungent smell of a salt marsh, or the fresh electric air right after a lightning storm.

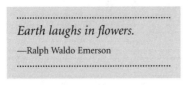

Earth laughs in flowers.
—Ralph Waldo Emerson

Even if it's raining, snowing, or dry as a drought—go outside, be fresh and real as nature itself. Because you are a part of nature yourself.

Keep On Keeping On

- Every day tell yourself: "This day, today, is new. It's another opportunity to feel good from being active."

- Variety is the spice of life. Do something different and fun every day.

- Allow joy into your life, in a physical way.

- Commit to moving just today. Avoid thinking about long-term commitments. Take it "one day at a time." Don't look at a whole week or month at a time; schedule your fun time for each day.

- Put some love and pleasure into it, every time. Think of how fun and good it is instead of focusing on how hard it is. (If it's too hard, don't do it.) Rephrase the old statement to become "Pain is no gain."

- Keep your expectations low. Exercise alone doesn't help you lose weight. (Eating less and exercise combined is what it takes.) Don't measure your results only in pounds—only gauge your progress by whether or not you were on your eating plan and were active *today*.

Getting started is the hardest part of being active. Once you do get active, joy is yours every day. We complete this chapter with a weekly activity log. Fill it out every day: write the day of the week, circle the amount of time in five minute intervals, and how you felt before and after. Increase the length of time by five minute intervals each week if you are able. Slowly build up to a minimum of thirty minutes daily over the course of one to two months. Do not go over sixty minutes. Make copies of this log, and fill them out every day!

THE JOY OF WEIGHT LOSS ACTIVITY LOG

DAY	TIME (minutes, increase weekly as able)						ACTIVITY	FEELINGS (before & after)
	5	10	15	20	25	30		
	5	10	15	20	25	30		
	5	10	15	20	25	30		
	5	10	15	20	25	30		
	5	10	15	20	25	30		
	5	10	15	20	25	30		
	5	10	15	20	25	30		

Part III: JOY ASSURED

You are going to be all right. Everything is going to come out fine in the end. You need have no fear of problems, your condition, or a wasted life. God is with you, in all ways, always. Your life is valuable. You are important, no matter what happens, because you are a child of God, an example of the creation of the One God. The Spirit of God is inside you, loving you, now. You and He are partners in living. Honor this life blessing by participating in your life, 100 percent. And thank God for your blessings; just to be alive at all! And for His love! Then you will always be fine.

You've Been OK All Along

> . . . love directed towards the eternal and infinite feeds the mind with pure joy, and is free from all sadness.
>
> —Benedict Spinoza

You didn't know it, but you've always been just fine. You have always been OK the way you were—perfect in your imperfections. God made you, and He wouldn't make anything that wasn't what He wanted. You've always been OK, the way that God wanted. You just didn't know it or believe it. You felt bad or ashamed about yourself and used extra food to feel better or to protect yourself from the pain of living. Furthermore, there was a snowball effect, because the worse you felt the more you ate, and the more you ate the worse you felt about gaining weight and feeling bad about yourself! Right?!

Get off the merry-go-round of self-hate, reframe your mind to be able to feel OK, and be self-assured because you're one of God's people. Make the conscious mental choice to now be OK, to now be with God. It's up to you to make up your mind to be physically, mentally, and spiritually *all right*.

The mind is the most important part of your weight loss success. You must train your mind to be free of its blocks, its fears and worries, its judgments of self-hatred and condemnation. In other words, you must let go of your troublesome mental constraints and begin to love yourself, because you love God.

You will find love in God. Think of God and surrender your problems over and over again. Train your mind toward love. Love is the subject over and over again. You get that love by loving God. You do that through an act of acknowledgement and surrender. Don't be afraid to give your problems up. I assure you, God is a very loving recipient!

Once you've surrendered your problems and begun to receive the divine assistance of love, God will liberate your history of poor eating and exercise habits and you'll be able to begin new habits. It all starts with your mind.

The idea here is to give your mind peace. To let God give you the feeling of safety and assurance in order to slowly and surely lose the weight and have a good life.

When you give your life to God, your peace, happiness, and joy is assured.

Why Concentrate on the Mind? Isn't Weight About the Body?

Your body is controlled by your mind. All of your desires, actions, and habits first originate in your mind. Even signals from the body—such as hunger, pain, hot, cold, fatigue, etc.—all go through your brain and are acted upon or not by the mind. To have a peaceful, fruitful, and joyous life it is essential that you train you mind and control your thoughts.

As humans, we are both blessed and cursed with an ability to form judgments and be aware of ourselves and our actions.

Self-awareness and consciousness are wonderful when they're loving, protective, and compassionate but are a real problem if you've somehow developed self-hatred, unnecessary fears and worries, or if they keep you from being your natural self. *If you use your conscious awareness to judge yourself negatively, this interrupts your natural cycles of change and adaptation.*

Each of us has natural cycles that must be lived; avoiding them or not allowing your cycles to occur leads to problems. Many of our

Unconsciously or subconsciously, we harbor what can become self-fulfilling prophecies—that our luck has run out, that we are prone to illness, that we have brought disease upon ourselves, that medicine can't cure everything, that doctors paint rosier pictures than may be merited, or that disability, loss of independence, suffering, or death are imminent.
That's why I have come to believe that faith in a bigger, stronger force is so influential.
—Herbert Benson, MD

"A psycho-neurosis must be understood as the suffering of a human being who has not discovered what life means for him. But all creativeness in the realm of the spirit as well as every psychic advance of man arises from a state of mental suffering, and it is spiritual stagnation, psychic sterility, which causes this state."
—Carl Jung

problems in life arise from negative self-judgments causing us to hold back, be blocked by fears, unable to cope, not participating in life, and allowing self-hatred to get the best of us.

We don't need to worry, however, because God has created us to be perfectly imperfect. What's funny is that it appears we're supposed to be blocked and have the self-hatred and interrupt our cycles, so we can have problems to work out by unblocking! God has evidently designed our minds so we can cycle between consciousness and unconsciousness, self-love and self-hatred (in the Freudian and Jungian sense of self-consciousness, negative conditioning and unconscious, hidden motivations and drives)! It seems almost automatic that we move forward in life, and then move backwards. It appears almost natural to have emotional blocks and self-doubts. As I see it our problems and pains, fears and blocks, joys and sorrows are actually blessings in disguise allowing us to overcome them with love and come to God for help! Our blindness and self-destructive habits are beautiful gifts that God has given us so we can surrender them, ask Him for help, and come to know His love, which was already there but to which we were blind! We really are OK; we just haven't thought we were. I hope you can truly appreciate this wonderful paradox and let it liberate you from your own self-imposed mental slavery.

Here's how to get off of the mental merry-go-round. In order to find the Joy of Weight Loss, try these:

Three Habits for Mental Liberation and Joyous Assurance

1. Be God's partner.

2. Actively participate in your life in every way, experiencing work and rest, sorrow and joy, pain and pleasure and then move on anew each day.

3. Be kind to yourself and practice compassion and empathy for all.

Let's take each one a little further:

1: BE GOD'S PARTNER

Know that it is impossible for you to be separate from God. While you are a unique individual, in the bigger sense of Creation you are a part of the whole. You are not at all alone; you are alive, here, a part of God and His Universe. *Until now, you only thought you were alone.* You didn't realize that God was always there, ready to be seen and to help. It's up to you to look and ask. It's up to you to accept the fact you are God's partner. You've been created for a purpose, whatever that purpose may be.

- Ask for God's help in every way, to know His plan for you, and to be able to put aside your blocks, fears, and self-hate.

- Surrender your painful desires to self-destruct through overeating and never moving.

- Ask for the ability and strength to create new habits and to be relieved of old destructive ones.

- Ask Him to give you the ability to stop eating when you are full.

- Ask Him to help you stop avoiding change and to know that transformation is inevitable and unavoidable.

- See God in all of your activites, in everything you do, and inside everyone you meet.

> *The intent of all commandments is that we acquire a firm belief in God, and proclaim Him as the One who has created us. This is, in fact, the very purpose of creation—for there is no other motive known to us. The Supreme Being asks of man only that he come to know Him and testify that He is the Creator. The prayers we recite, the synagogues we build, the convocations we hold—all are designed to give outward expression to our inner conviction that He is our Creator. We assemble in the House of Prayer and cry out: We are Your creations!*
> —Ramban

Here's a very powerful and very helpful habit to acquire that will help you know that you're not alone, that you are a valuable part of God's creation, and let you develop comfort and joy in being God's partner. See God in everything and in everyone.

Everything you do, say to yourself: **"I Do This for God."**
Everything you see, say to yourself: **"That's a Part of God."**
Everyone you encounter, say to yourself: **"There Is God in Them, Too."**

If you look for the truth outside yourself, it gets farther and farther away. Today, walking alone, I meet him everywhere I step. He is the same as me, yet I am not him. Only if you understand it in this way will you merge with the way things are.

—Tung-Shan (807–869)

This will quickly give you an incredible Godhead high! The illusion you're holding on to, that you are alone and separate, unimportant, invisible, unable, unworthy, and ugly will soon disappear in a profoundly wonderful, joyous sea of God's love. Practice this habit for the rest of your life, and you will be forever joyous.

Armed with this enlightenment and spiritual bliss, you will then easily acknowledge and actually appreciate your fears, shame, humility, and worries, be able to put them aside, and rise above them with the warmth of God's spiritual love and care for you. You will then, easily, do what you need to do. God will guide you and never let you fail, even though you may yet again forget these spiritual truths and revert to old habits. If that occurs, just surrender and acknowledge Him again, and then you'll be fine: because you are in partnership with God.

2: PARTICIPATE IN LIFE 100 PERCENT

Eating is never so simple as hunger.

—Erica Jong

Now that you're with God, there's nothing that can harm you. Just dive into life! Put your desires to be better and your belief in the power of God into action. There's no need to hold back anymore.

- If you truly want to lose weight and be healthier, pay attention to these desires and act on them. Follow the Joy of Weight Loss Eating and Activity plans and do your best to eat healthily. Be active: Just go out and get going every day and learn to love it. It'll happen, just do it!

- Go ahead and make mistakes. You're supposed to! You learn from them! God is there to help you, and with Him you cannot ever ultimately fail, nor will your soul ever be harmed or diminished in any way. Get hurt (but not too badly, of course), wear yourself thin, use yourself up—that's why you're here!

- Go ahead and experience the range and depth of your emotions: allowing yourself to be yourself, feeling the sorrow and pain and talking about it, never holding it in or preventing it from being.

- Then let go of the feelings and get over the problem. Let your troubles naturally change course; they always will in time. Never attach or cling to problems; let them go away after you've used them for learning.

Here are two more active, positive habits that will help you achieve the Joy of Weight Loss…

Differentiate Between Hunger or Habit

A lot of us folks with histories of weight problems have lost the ability to feel the natural hunger feeling. Some of us (like me) never experienced it at all, because we were always overeating and never felt true hunger. It's OK and healthy to allow yourself to be a little hungry. It's not OK to be extremely hungry or go more than two to four hours between eating.

- Hunger originates in the stomach and is a "body" sensation. Sometimes it feels like a slight weakness, euphoria, emerging headache, shakiness, a "gnawing" in the gut, or a real bodily emptiness. To a small degree, these are all normal, healthy feelings!

- Habits are in the head and heart. We think we're hungry or we're bored or feeling emotionally unhappy or needy. We may have just eaten and still think we're hungry when we're actually not. If this happens to you, you need to ask yourself when you last ate. If it was less than two hours ago, the hungry feeling is probably a habit talking and not real hunger. Ask yourself how you are feeling right at that moment and take time to think and feel if you are truly hungry.

- Feel safe with God and break the millions of connections (conscious and unconscious) that trigger eating when you're not actually hungry. Refer to the food logs you're about to write in the Daily Companion in order to spot habit patterns and "trigger" connections. And don't expect to do this immediately. You have the rest of your life to do it!

The Feeling of Enough

Another God-given mechanism in us, that many weight strugglers have either never experienced or learned to override long ago, is the instinctual feeling of "enough." It's a very subtle kind of internal knowledge that you're satisfied, even though you may not have eaten everything on your plate or what you're supposed to eat. It comes fairly quietly and only when you're in the middle of eating or twenty minutes after you've eaten your servings and gotten up from the table, if you are a speedy eater. Look and listen for it, and make sure to honor and follow it, because it's a real gift of God's guidance.

- Learn to spot your subtle "enough" feeling.

- Take a deep breath, close your eyes, and say a prayer for the power to stop the instant you feel it.

- Receive Divine grace and stopping power, and honor God by doing it.

- Get up from the table and away from the food. If you're at a restaurant, ask the waiter to take the food away and wrap it to go for tomorrow. Or go to the restroom to wash your hands. Or brush your teeth. Or call a friend on the phone and tell them what's happening. That lapse in time will joyously distract you from having to overeat.

- If you must remain with the food, make it ugly and inedible—put your napkin over it, dump an ashtray on it, mix it with too much ketchup or mustard so it's disgusting. (This "playing with your food" is another source of joy!)

- If you've completed your meal and eaten your allocated servings but aren't yet feeling you've had "enough," wait twenty minutes from the time when you finished for your stomach to tell your brain that you are satisfied. It takes that long sometimes, but it will always come if you wait. (This is an actual metabolic activity. Your stomach secretes a chemical called tryptophane upon being sufficiently filled, which takes twenty minutes to get to your brain. The brain then tells your system: "Enough! Stop eating now!")

Participate in Life

- If you don't have one already, get into a hobby—something that will employ your mind and hands. Be creative: Build things like arts and crafts projects, get into gardening, or home decorating, home canning, caring for animals, playing a musical instrument, drawing or painting, sewing or knitting, investing, or collecting and restoring antiques. Play challenging games: chess, crossword puzzles, trivia quizzes, cards, logic puzzles, computer games. A hobby will not only connect you with your latent talents and give you new friends, it will sharpen your mind.

- Join a club, whether it's for: readers, philosophers, square dancers, artists, writers, horticulturists, climbers; those who enjoy racquet sports, basketball, music, theater, real estate, textiles, fashion, discount shopping, travel, woodworking, spiritual study, concert-going; women's groups, men's groups, civic, social, and professional groups.

- Volunteer your time: hospitals, charities, hospices, children, school PTA, libraries, community recreation centers, conservancies, museums, social assistance agencies, homeless aid, veterinary shelters, and clinics all need people to help. Doing this will give you a great sense of joy and accomplishment.

3: PRACTICE KINDNESS, EMPATHY, AND COMPASSION

> "My religion is very simple. My religion is kindness."
> —His Holiness, The Dalai Lama

Be kind to yourself at all times. Give yourself the benefit of your doubt. Be your own best friend, because you'll never have a better one than you. Do not repress any thought or emotion you have and don't hold on to any thought or feeling for too long. Let your thoughts and feelings flow; take action on the ones that are going to help you; and let every other one go by without attachment. You do have the power to do this, and you're free to exercise it.

Whenever you are feeling down, or in sorrow or pain, offer yourself some relief. Tell yourself that it's OK to feel blue; that this feeling, like all others before, will pass." Tell yourself that you're going to be OK. It's true, you will be just fine no matter what may come because of God's love and forgiveness for you.

I've found God to be amazingly kind and understanding. When I am doing my best—meaning well, trying to be a good person, trying to understand and follow God's direction—even though I make mistakes, they seem to be purposeful. It's as if, for me, I needed some pain and unpleasantness in order to be motivated to do something different. But God is compassionate and kind, in that the hardship I experience is never more than I can tolerate or learn to cope with. This compassion is what lets me go on living. Without it, I'd have been dead a long time ago!

Be kind and compassionate with your weight loss and management, and your life:

- Take your time and go slowly. You have the rest of your long life to become what you want and need to be. In terms of weight loss, take it slowly and only lose one to two pounds a week, over time. Any more and, so experts believe, it could be harmful. It's OK for you not to lose or even gain a little weight from time to time. It's the overall, long-term change you're looking for, not the weekly, daily, or even hourly fluctuations you will encounter. Once they've reached their reasonable weight point, most people who manage their weight keep it within a range of five pounds up or down. If you're over five pounds up or down, then you can gradually modify your food and activity to adjust. Nothing extreme. It's not an emergency. Just be mindful.

- Set a *reasonable* weight goal between you, God, and your doctor. Do not base your weight on any insurance or pharmaceutical company charts, which may be unrealistic for you. Take your family history into account, as well as age, level of fitness, and vital statistics—such as condition of your heart, lungs, and major organs as reviewed by your physician. Perhaps you don't even need to lose weight at all, or just a little will be enough to get you healthier.

- Set new personal weight standards and benchmarks: clothing size, how you feel and move, flexibility and muscle tone, and your overall health, instead of just pounds or inches. Lose the obsession along with the weight.

- If you're still into the pounds and inches (and I don't actually know anyone who isn't to varying degrees!), *weigh yourself only once a month, at the same day and time,* preferably before you've swallowed anything that day and with no clothes on. Write your weight down on a little piece of paper. Better yet, measure three areas: waist, thighs, and breast. Note your clothing sizes. Record those figures once a month as well.

- Never do anything that doesn't feel right. Pay attention to your instincts and let your conscience be your guide. More often than not, it's your first impression that's correct.

- When it comes to eating, choose what you're hungry for, making sure it's an instinctual hunger and not a habit. I believe that our bodies provide signals to us, and it's important to listen and serve them. If you're craving protein, have some lower-fat fish or poultry, beans or a few nuts. If you crave dairy, it may be you need calcium—so have some milk, cheese, or yogurt. If vegetables seem to hit the spot, by all means have some. Same goes for fruit if you want some sweets.

With Appreciation

Give yourself and God lots of praise. As long as you're doing your best, you deserve a lot of praise and respect. Just for giving you life, and keeping you alive, doesn't God deserve a lot of thanks?

> *i found god in myself and i loved her i loved her fiercely.*
> —Ntozake Shange

- Every morning, as you wake up, let your first thought be one of gratitude to God. Appreciate your existence and the good things that have been given to you by your maker. Don't get stuck on what you don't have or what you want. Surrender your problems and commit to improving things.

- Every morning, take time to appreciate yourself. Count your blessings. See the bright side. Acknowledge what's good in your life. Sort out the most important things you need to do today, and do only them: connecting to God, caring for your family, enjoying your work, eating in moderation, and being active.

- Take time for some silent reflection and meditation every morning after you've showered and dressed but before you begin your day. Just one minute or five minutes is enough, or if there's time, ten, twenty, even thirty minutes are marvelously helpful. Just go to a private place, close your eyes, be quiet, and be still. Let any thoughts that come float silently away. Just let yourself "be," silently, consciously, peacefully.

Be Kind To Others

As you want others to be kind and good to you, be the same to them. Practice seeing God in everyone and in everything. Realize that when you give someone your attention and care, you are really giving it to God, inside them. This means that by *being loving to others, you're being loving to your deepest self at the same time*, because the same God is in all of us! This is a profoundly important realization. If everyone knew and practiced this awesome truth, there would be no problems in the world.

Agape

Dr. Harville Hendrix and his wife and partner Helen LaKelly Hunt, who wrote the foreword to this book and the definitive guide to love and empathy in relationships and marriage called *Getting the Love You Want*, taught me that empathy and care for others was called *agape* in Greek, and I think it's the true definition of love. Agape means seeing God in others and in yourself, and treating your fellow man and woman with love because of it.

How does one practice agape, empathy, and compassion for others?

- Begin by really taking the time to listen to people. Put your own thoughts and needs aside for a moment (they'll be there when you're done, don't worry).

- As you listen, understand where the other person is coming from. Feel their pain. Make an effort to experience the other person's joys and sorrows from their perspective.

- Offer your help in a way that you feel able to, and in the exact way the person wants to be helped. Don't give people what you think they need; give them what they say they need. In doing this, I've learned you're actually healing yourself and the other person at the same time (according to Hendrix and Hunt).

- Realize the other person is a human being, just like you are, with feelings, cares, needs, talents, defects, and the need to love and be loved.

Four ❧

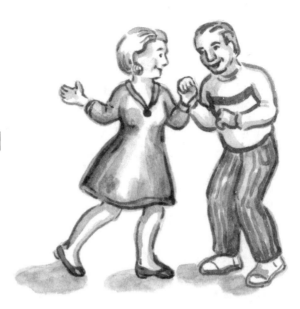

Joy, Continued

Joyous living—being able to cope with your problems and free of excess weight for the rest of your life—is the goal of this book and your life. To be free of the weight problem once and for all, simply keep on doing all of the positive work you have been doing. Ultimately your goal should be to completely integrate all the new habits, the different ways of thinking about food and activity, the commitment to action, the spiritual surrender and love, and the feeling of assurance into your life. That's a lot to do! But you can do it, if you take it slowly and consistently.

You don't do this all at once: it takes time. Often it takes months or years just to get started. That's OK; you have time, so please take it. You did not put on the extra weight all at once, it took awhile; therefore let it take time to get it off, and give it your time and attention on a daily basis to maintain what you have lost.

This is a program for life, because it is about lifestyle changes. Unlike diets that you start and stop, this plan is one that you stick with. It's not a temporary fix, a remedy, or a cure—*the joy of weight loss is a way of life.* You just keep doing what works for you, in ways you can live with.

The serious problems in life are never fully solved. If ever they should appear so it is a sure sign that something has been lost. The meaning and purpose of a problem seem to lie not in its solution but in our working at it incessantly. This alone preserves us from stultification and petrification.
—Carl Jung

Hopefully, you've read the earlier chapters of this book and have begun to think about and actually tried some of the suggestions. You've learned to allow yourself both joy and sorrow and to let go of your urge to repress difficult and painful feelings. You've realized you were creating your own problem (unintentionally) and have freed yourself of the burden by asking God for help. Now it's a matter of just going on, dealing and coping, and trying your best. You've learned what and how to eat normally and in moderation. You've begun to move again, at your own pace, and to find enjoyment in being active.

Don't stop now! You're on the right track! Keep trying! Things are changing for the better.

The Great Stumbling Block

As hard as you may try, and as much as you want to succeed deep down, you may be encountering some internal blocks. Something inside keeps you from actually doing what you want or need to do. Some hidden force prevents you from eating properly, stops you from getting up and out the door to move your body. Some inner mystery keeps you sitting, overeating, in front of the TV or cramming junk food into your mouth, or over-consuming at restaurants.

To get over this mystery blockage forever, you need to uncover it, begin to accept it, and actually learn to love living with it.

You will, of course, need to do your own detective work to find exactly what it is in you that sabotages your success: what causes it, what started it, why you're holding on to it, and why it is so dangerous to let go of it. Each person's blocks, histories, and mysteries are unique.

What you need to understand is that this blockage is fiercely guarded by your inner mind. It's buried in the deepest, most inaccessible part of you. It can take lots of intense work in therapy to even get close to it. It's valuable to know what your emotional blocks are, why they occur, and what purpose they may serve as long as you do it to ultimately rise above these blocks and stop their control over you. You may also uncover and learn to live with your blocks and saboteurs by participating in life as completely as possible. Life itself teaches you about your blocks. If you can understand and rise above them, and even come to appreciate their necessity and service to you, then your life truly will be joyous.

26 Behold the fowls of the air: for they sow not, neither do they reap, nor gather into barns: yet your heavenly Father feedeth them. Are ye not much better than they?

27 Which of you by taking thought can add one cubit unto his stature?

28 And why take ye thought for raiment? Consider the lilies of the field, how they grow; they toil not, neither do they spin:

29 And yet I say unto you, That even Solomon in all his glory was not arrayed like one of these.

30 Wherefore, if God so clothe the grass of the field, which to day is, and tomorrow is cast into the oven, shall he not much more clothe you, O ye of little faith?

31 Therefore take no thought, saying, What shall we eat? or, What shall we drink? or, Wherewithal shall we be clothed?

32 (For after all these things, do the Gentiles seek:) for your heavenly Father knoweth that ye have need of all these things.

33 But seek ye first the kingdom of God, and his righteousness; and all these things shall be added unto you.

34 Take therefore no thought for the morrow: for the morrow shall take thought for the things of itself…

—The Holy Bible, Matthew 6

It often takes a lifetime of experiences to begin to even see yourself clearly, much less deal with your problems. Why, you may ask, do you have this block, this hindrance that prevents you from being your best?

All I can say is that something that is so deep and powerfully controlling in your life must be important in some way. You must need your blocks and self-destructive behaviors in order to function. This may seem incredible to you: that you might need the weight, the overeating, the inactivity, the fears and self-hatred. It's a paradox, one that I admit I don't fully understand. But I believe that God must have given us these blocks, problems, fears, and painful self-criticisms to give us something to work on, something to accomplish.

The truth is your blocks define your personality. You only *think* they're problems. You think your being overweight or obese is negative, when actually you needed to be that way. You needed the suffering, anxiety, and fear. You protected yourself with it. You eased your pain a little with the self-destructive over-consumption. You felt empty and lost, you bore a lot of pain and suffering and kept it under wraps. You survived.

Rise Above and Become Conscious

It is impossible to erase your blocks. I suggest that you stop trying to kill off that part of you that's preventing you from living fully, to cease feeling bad about feeling bad! Your blocks are the fabric of your soul that you and God have woven together in order for you to be you, and to live.

All you need to do is be aware that your blocks and pain are there for a purpose. They once served you well, even though now that purpose is over—revealed, exposed, known, even understood and loved. You were supposed to go through what you've been through, and now you're evidently supposed to move onto the next phase of your life.

Use the technique of "rising above." When you're feeling down, blue, in emotional pain, or desperate for some comfort and joy…

1. Acknowledge your feelings. Try to clearly see what's upsetting you. Know that it will not usually be logical (that's a different part of you).

2. Get to the need. Ask yourself: "What do I truly need from this feeling?" It may be that you just need someone to listen, or some affection, or to take a little time to sort out the feelings and needs (often that's enough in itself).

3. Consciously *rise above* the feelings and needs. Use the higher, more aware part of your mind to both *acknowledge* and *act* on the situation.
   a. You could get the need met. Ask another person to listen to you or give you some affection. Tell God your problems and ask for help. Give yourself what you need: time in the day for yourself, a favor from a friend, a good conversation, a hug, a walk in the woods or that book or CD you've wanted.
   b. You could decide to let it be and move on. Not every feeling and need requires attention or action. Often, no reaction at all is the best course of action. It may be that you're just going to feel bad for a while, and that's OK! Time will pass and you have the ability to cope.

If you can develop these skills, this is a strong sign of stability and maturity. It's a bold act of self-love as well; to allow yourself to feel and experience, then consciously rise above, your feelings and deal with them in constructive, positive ways.

The Right Track

The ingredients for your complete, joyful weight loss are in this book. They're all you need. Just keep doing them, one day at a time, and you will know the joy of weight loss slowly over time. To recap:

- Accept and appreciate your pain and sorrow. Let it be and then let it go, and allow the joy that's embedded within the pain and sorrow to radiate forth.

- Surrender your problems, fears, and sorrows to God all day, every day. Then surrender your joy, happiness, and fulfillment to Him, in grateful appreciation for your life.

- Eat a range of healthy foods and what you like in moderation. Stay with a structured eating plan but be free to have what you like within that structure. Refer to the "Joy of Eating Continuation Plan" below.

- Be joyously active every day. Build up to the goal of thirty minutes of moderate activity every day, or more. Refer to the "Joyous Activity Continuation Plan" below.

- Be assured. Know that you are important and cared about by God and by all of us who have been through or are going through similar challenges in our lives. Find someone to care about; share yourself; help them to know what you know; and do what you're doing together.

To maintain your weight loss victory and stay healthy, you need to be active every day. The best way to do that is to *continue surrendering your old habits and preconceptions to God and integrate daily physical activity into your lifestyle.*

Get started. You just get into it. Once you start, it's enjoyable; the hardest part is to get started. Do it every day, consistently.

Once you've begun, you'll quickly realize that if you don't move and stay active every day, you feel really bad. Fitness takes weeks or months of consistent daily participation to develop, but only one week to lose. When you lose your level of fitness, you instantly know it from achy joints and tight, stiff muscles, sore back, neck, or shoulders, a loss of energy, and eventually more frequent sickness and diseases. God gave us all incentives to remain active and be joyous!

The Joy of Weight Loss Continuation Plan

The idea is just to continue the way you've been eating when you were losing weight, but now you may slowly, experimentally increase your number of servings, in order to maintain your weight at a stable level within +/- five pounds per month. You may slowly add more servings per day, which means slightly more food overall. You may also add an occasional dessert or snack food, ideally one per week, asking God to help you refrain from compulsive overeating. Continue to limit fatty, salty or sweet foods, but you may have some—as long as you don't forget they have a lot of "empty" calories. You've changed your eating lifestyle, and learned new consumption habits: keep it up, one day at a time, for the rest of your life.

1. Always, before eating, stop and allow yourself a feeling of joy and appreciation. Take a moment of silence to value yourself, the food, and God.
2. Make sure you're enjoying your eating: the occasion, the sustenance, anyone you're with, and the bounty and blessings you're receiving.
3. Be sure to have foods from all six USDA Food Pyramid groups every day. *Have three meals per day and three snacks per day or three larger meals and one snack a day,* each consisting of:

   • **Protein (from both dairy and meat groups)**

   • **Grain**

   • **Fruits and/or Vegetables (having both groups each day)**

Active Women
(and most men)

You may *slowly* increase the number of servings* overall per day, monitoring your weight on a monthly basis, up to:

GRAINS: nine servings per day

VEGETABLES: four servings per day

FRUITS: three servings per day

DAIRY: two to three servings per day (teenagers, young adults to age twenty-four, pregnant or breast-feeding women need three a day)

PROTEIN: Two servings a day from the meat/nuts/beans group (six ounces of lean meat)

Active Men

You may slowly increase the number of servings* overall per day, monitoring your weight on a monthly basis, up to:

GRAINS: eleven servings per day

VEGETABLES: five servings per day

FRUITS: four servings per day

DAIRY: two to three servings per day (teenagers, young adults to age twenty-four, need three a day)

PROTEIN: three servings per day from the meat/nuts/beans group (seven ounces total)

- **DRINK a large glass of water (eight to ten ounces) with every meal and snack, for a minimum of six glasses daily.**

- **WAIT twenty minutes after you finish eating, in order to feel full. You will feel full. Give it time!**

- **STOPPING POWER: Say a prayer to God, asking for help to stop when you've had enough. Then leave the table.**

* Based on the USDA Food Guide Pyramid/Dietary Guidelines for Americans, 2000.

To sum up everything I've been saying to you in a variety of ways, the joy of weight loss is something you choose to give yourself. You make a conscious choice, not just once, but thousands of times a day to forego temporary pleasure and pain in the service of lasting joy.

Every time you try to experience your full, honest range of emotions and deal with them—experiencing some pain, suffering, and sorrow yet eventually letting go and coping in spite of the hardship—you are choosing joy.

Each time you rise above your problems—letting go and surrendering them to God, admitting you cannot do it all alone—you are choosing joy.

When you stop eating after you've had the right amount of servings, when you eat from all food groups in small amounts, and when you do not stuff yourself for immediate pleasure and self-gratification—you are choosing joy.

When each day you get out and enjoy being active, even though you don't feel like it or are embarrassed at first—you are choosing joy.

The Joyous Activity Continuation Plan

- **A minimum of thirty minutes daily of moderate activity: walking, dancing, swimming, racquet sports, golf, housework, fishing, bicycling, canoeing, home improvement. Or more vigorous activities such as aerobics, cardiovascular conditioning, running or jogging, water or snow sports, gardening, or competitive sports, etc.**

- **Ideally, work up to sixty minutes per day, either in one session, or divided into whatever is convenient. But do not go for more than sixty minutes on any given day.**

- **Vary activities day by day (as I do), making them a part of your life.**

Choose a schedule that you can keep by including it each day, and love doing it, for example:

THE FIVE-DAY-A-WEEK WORKER ACTIVITY SCHEDULE

Monday through Friday: Thirty minutes of moderate activity like walking either to/from work, at lunch, right after work; thirty minutes of moderate activity like swimming, dancing, golf, home improvement, etc. either before or after work; or three twenty-minute sessions, or six ten-minute sessions.

Weekends: Sixty minutes per day playing sports, aerobic classes, boxing, bicycling, etc.

THE EVERY OTHER DAY FREELANCER ACTIVITY SCHEDULE

Monday–Wednesday–Friday: Thirty minutes of very active or vigorous physical activity like aerobics, jogging, tennis, etc. (Take classes!)

Tuesday–Thursday–Saturday–Sunday: Sixty minutes daily of moderate activity like walking, dancing, swimming, racquet sports, golf, housework, home improvement, etc.

THE MIX-AND-MATCH AS YOU LIKE IT ACTIVITY SCHEDULE

This is the one that I do, integrating it into my life and loving it. Vary it day by day, week by week, but be sure to be active (moderate or vigorous) every day.

MONDAY: Racquetball, tennis or squash with a family member, co-worker or friend

TUESDAY: Early morning dance aerobics class, one hour

WEDNESDAY: Swimming, one hour

THURSDAY: Early morning dance aerobics class, one hour

FRIDAY: Walking to work, and back, thirty to sixty minutes each way

SATURDAY: Hiking in the woods, one hour

SUNDAY: A stroll through the mall, all afternoon

Five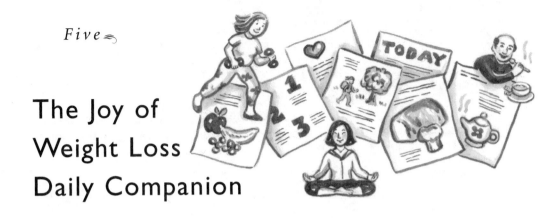

The Joy of Weight Loss Daily Companion

A Thirty-Day Personal Guide

This is a day-by-day, sequential guide that will help you get healthier and happier and personally experience the joy of weight loss. Follow its ideas, suggestions, and activities, faithfully doing them a little at a time, day by day. Your mind will change and your body will follow.

Please feel free to refer to the first four chapters of this book. They are there to completely teach you the ideas and methods of what you will find here in a more abbreviated form. Do the work day by day. It's only a little effort that's required, little by little, on all levels of your life: spiritual, mental, and physical. Let me be your daily guide and let God be your companion and inspiration as you change your attitudes, beliefs, and lifestyle. Think the thoughts, eat the food, move your body, express and release your emotions! Do it, without delay. Do it without ceasing.

Give this program at least one month. I promise you that if you make the slightest effort and do what I ask of you each day, you will succeed, the weight loss will happen, your mind will be open and refreshed, your soul fed, and your relationship with God solid. At the end of the month, you will have integrated healthy eating patterns into your life and will be meeting the minimum suggested amounts of physical activity every day. Most of all, you'll be enjoying the process of a healthy, happy life.

Day One

TODAY'S JOYOUS THOUGHT: *Congratulations!*

You have taken the first step. You have begun your life anew. Congratulations. It may not seem like much, but what you've done is actually rather wonderful. You've made a conscious choice to work on a problem you're experiencing. In doing something about that problem, you've also acknowledged that the problem exists. For that you deserve a lot or praise.

You could have just done nothing. You could have just continued the old habits, felt the pain of overweight, gone ahead and felt bad about it but continued to overeat. Instead, you did something. You've come to the right place. Keep up the good work. You can do this, because it's not that hard if you take it piece by piece and learn the real truth about weight loss.

DO THIS TODAY: *See Joy*

Today, like every day, I want you to do something purposeful for yourself. Today, I'd like you to see the joy in at least one thing you do or in something about yourself. Bonne, a young woman with a former weight problem who is in my television and video special, felt really bad. She was fifty pounds overweight and very unhappy. When I encouraged her to find something about herself that made her joyful, she was able to see that she had great legs! "I have my mother's legs," she said, "muscular, shapely, good." Even though she was not happy about the rest of her body, she was able to change her thinking at least to find one positive thing. She referred to her great legs over and over again, made small changes and didn't give up, and has now lost the fifty pounds forever.

What's something of joy that you do or have? Do you have good legs or a pretty smile, or are you a caring, good person? Perhaps you have a good job or career, or a nice home, spouse, family, and friends. See if you can come up with a list. Count your blessings today.

Until one is committed, there is hesitancy, the chance to draw back, always ineffectiveness. Concerning all acts of initiative and creation, there is one elementary truth the ignorance of which kills countless ideas and splendid plans: that the moment one definitely commits oneself, then providence moves too. All sorts of things occur to help one that would never otherwise have occurred. A whole stream of events issues from the decision, raising in one's favor all manner of unforeseen incidents, meetings and material assistance which no man could have dreamed would have come his way. Whatever you can do or dream you can, begin it. Boldness has genius, power and magic in it. Begin it now.
—Johann Wolfgang von Goethe

TODAY'S MENU AND ACTIVITY:

Also, today, like every day, I want you to do one little thing about your eating. Don't worry, it'll be a source of joy if you will only do the one little thing each day. Trust me!

Today, I'd like you to write down everything you put in your mouth: what time, where, how much, what you were doing, and how you felt just before and after you ate it. Don't change a thing. Do not try to diet or eat less. Just eat the way you would normally eat or overeat. This idea is for you to become aware of some things about yourself. Be honest: no one will see this but you (and God, of course!).

I also want you to write what movement, activity, or exercise you've done today. Anytime, any way you moved your body. Write all of this down here. If you need more space, use another piece of paper.

PRAYER AND MEDITATION

Sit for five minutes in silence, with your eyes closed, taking slow, methodical deep breaths. Clear your mind of all thoughts, and mentally say to yourself with each in and out breath: "I Am." (What this does is to ground you, to enable you to feel both your presence and God's presence inside of you, helping you.)

WHAT FOOD/ ACTIVITY	TIME	WHERE	AMOUNTS (in cups)	DOING WHAT (while eating)	FEELINGS (before/after)

Day Two

TODAY'S JOYOUS THOUGHT: *Intentional Joy*

Becoming happy doesn't just happen. Joy doesn't just come for nothing! You have to set the stage. You have to be involved in life, actively participating, expressing, feeling, and being. For joy to come to you, you have to look for it in places where you wouldn't expect it. It takes opening a different side of yourself and making an effort to see the positive and not just the negative in any given situation or feeling. You have to invest in the possibility that you can have a joyous life and then set about finding it.

An example of looking for joy in weight loss is to discover the difference between pleasure and joy. Pleasure is a temporary feeling of satisfaction, a short-term high, a "rush," a "quick-fix" of comfort you get from overeating. Pleasure doesn't last long, and it has a lot of side effects like being over-stuffed and obese. Joy, on the other hand, is a long-term feeling without any side effects at all! You get it from structured eating, being active, having a connection to nature, God, and other people, and through healthy living.

DO THIS TODAY: *Uncovering Joy*

Look for joy where you least expect it: In someone's smile, a beautiful flower, helping another person in need, seeing past your own suffering to understand someone else's, a job well done, being patient, the quality of the color blue, a whiff of spring or fall in the air, a neatly pressed shirt, not having another helping.

> *Life does not need comfort, when it can be offered meaning, nor pleasure, when it can be shown purpose. Reveal what is the purpose of existence and how he may attain it—the steps he must take—and man will go forward again hardily, happily, knowing that he has found what he must have—intentional living—and knowing that an effort, which takes all his energy because it is worth his full and constant concentration, is the only life deserving the devotion, satisfying the nature, and developing the potentialities of a self-conscious being.*
>
> —Anonymous

TODAY'S MENU AND ACTIVITY

Again, just keep doing what you're doing, and keep written track of it. Take joy in being meticulous!

WHAT FOOD/ ACTIVITY	TIME	WHERE	AMOUNTS (in cups)	DOING WHAT (while eating)	FEELINGS (before/after)

PRAYER AND MEDITATION: *Opening Your Heart*

In a quiet place, such as your bedroom, lay down, close your eyes, and be quiet for five minutes. Notice your breath flowing in and out. Clear your mind of as many thoughts as possible, letting each one just drift away. Luxuriate in this moment, this private time that is all yours. After five minutes, slowly let your mind come back into the world, and think of a time when you felt joy. Maybe it was when you had a new friend, when someone gave you something really special, or when somebody took the time to listen to you or help you. Picture how good you felt. Let all of the feelings come in. Go ahead and feel the wholeness of the memory. Now, after another five minutes or so, be cleansed and relieved after having had the luxury of feeling. With eyes still closed, imagine your heart has a locked door. See that door clearly, then at the right moment open the doorway to your heart, allowing joy to come into your life, today.

Day Three

TODAY'S JOYOUS THOUGHT: *Details*

They say that God is in the details. I think that's true. I also say "joy is in the details," as well. Details are necessary parts of the whole—the little points, the peculiarities, the pieces of the puzzle. Without them, there is no whole.

Keeping track of your foods and activities is detail work. It may seem like a bit of a burden, but it's a necessary pain. Though it's still too early to spot any patterns you may have, your logs will, ultimately, be very useful after a week's worth of efforts. The more detail-oriented and precise you are about keeping the logs, the deeper your understanding of your habit patterns. When you look back, you will find a great deal of joy in these details. You may even find God in them!

DO THIS TODAY: *Good Measure*

Just by keeping logs of what I ate and did, how, where, when, why and what I felt, I actually lost weight. I did nothing different, I just became consciously aware of things. Just doing that helped me lose weight.

Today, I want you to really get detail-oriented. Get obsessed with measuring. If you aren't already using a measuring cup to help keep your logs, by all means get one and use it. Also, a dietary scale would be useful for weighing cereals and meats (don't be afraid of the word dietary, it means "what you eat" here!). Measure every morsel you put on your plate, every tidbit you put in your mouth. Time your physical activities with a stopwatch or wristwatch, log the start and end times. Count everything and make the count count!

TODAY'S MENU AND ACTIVITY

Again, for today, keep those logs. This time, be yet more precise and actually measure the amount of everything.

WHAT FOOD/ ACTIVITY	TIME	WHERE	AMOUNTS (in cups)	DOING WHAT (while eating)	FEELINGS (before/after)

PRAYER AND MEDITATION

Find, again, a private sanctuary where you can be quiet and by yourself. Collect your thoughts and take five minutes to be still and totally peaceful.

Say a prayer to God, in your own way, in your own words. Something like: "God, I want to find new ways. I want to be open to seeing things differently. I want to embrace new methods and not shy away from becoming better and experiencing my life anew. I give you my fear and hesitations. I give you my blocks and limitations. I ask that you grant me the ability to get totally involved in the details of change."

Day Four

TODAY'S JOYOUS THOUGHT: *Remembering*

Was there a time when you didn't have a weight problem—a time when you didn't think about what you were eating, never feeling guilty or self-judging, not worried about getting enough exercise because you were so active? Think back to that time. Remember what it was like to be free of excesses in your life: excess food, weight, worry, shame. Is this memory happy, mixed, or unpleasant? Do you feel joy in this memory of being lighter or is there sadness mixed in?

DO THIS TODAY: *Let Your Emotions Be Whole*

Take time to think of joyous times. Remember what it was like to just be yourself, not tied to weight and self-esteem sufferings. Feel the memory of liberation, of being unaware of problems. If you begin to feel sad afterwards because you miss that time, or you're full of sorrow because you're getting older, or if you miss someone or something that you no longer have—go ahead and let yourself feel it. Just let whatever thought and emotion you have happen; don't hold it back anymore. Open up and let it in, and know that every joy has a sorrow behind it. Realize that in order to feel the joy of living, you must also accept and nurture the sorrow along with it and then move on. If you can get good at doing this, becoming real and whole in your emotional life, then you will begin to experience a lifting up, a kind of relief, a sense of freedom. And then joy will really be yours.

TODAY'S MENU AND ACTIVITY

Guess what? Another day of logging! You're half-way through. Make sure you measure and write down everything, filling in every blank. If you forget, then go back later and write it down.

WHAT FOOD/ ACTIVITY	TIME	WHERE	AMOUNTS (in cups)	DOING WHAT (while eating)	FEELINGS (before/after)

PRAYER AND MEDITATION: *Sweet Sorrow*

Take five minutes for silent meditation. Then say this prayer.

"God, let me be able to feel all my emotions. Let me experience both the joy and the sorrow, the bitter and the sweet. If it be your will, allow me to be myself in every way, unhampered by feelings that are too painful to let surface."

Day Five

TODAY'S JOYOUS THOUGHT: *Overcoming Inertia and Expectations*

There's a law of physics—Isaac Newton's as a matter of fact—that says it takes more energy to get started than it does to keep something going. It's called "overcoming inertia." You have to push harder to start a ball rolling. The same is true if you want to lose weight. You have to give it a little extra push. Once you lose the weight, then it takes less effort to keep the change going. This is something to look forward to.

Starting up, you have to get over the hurdle of mental inertia. The blockage of mind, the thoughts and beliefs that keep you the way you are. It first takes giving up any expectations you have about how to lose weight, and how your life may be different if you do. It takes a mental effort to start the process of bodily change—a detailed, structured, constant effort. But you can do it. You've already started.

DO THIS TODAY: *Give Up the Expectations*

Here is another truth: you are causing your own weight problem because you're holding on to old ideas, self-hatred, fears, desires, and expectations. I go into this more thoroughly in the second and fourth chapters, which I encourage you to re-read. Right now, I'd like to suggest that you just give up any expectations you may have. From here on, every time you think you know how to "diet" or what foods to eat and how much, forget them. They didn't serve you well in the past, and they won't work now. Give up the thought that you can be perfectly thin, too, while you are at it. You will probably never be perfect or perfectly thin. (Healthy, yes; reasonable, sound; safe weight, definitely yes. Beautiful and sexy, absolutely! But perfect? No!) Give up the belief that you have to exercise intensely every day. You simply do not in order to be healthier. Yes, you need to move and be active, but doing so can be simple and joyous and you'll accomplish a lot. Finally, today, give up the concept that if you lose weight, you will be happy and your whole life will be great. The truth is, you need to get happy now and make your whole life great, then you will lose the weight. If you just lose a lot, with expectations of being a different person but making no change in your thoughts and beliefs, you will be in for a major shock. You'll still be the same, unhappy, and miserable person, just thinner, that's all. Believe me, I've been there and done that! So wipe your expectation slate clean, today and every day. Put your expectations aside, every time they come up, and just stick with the Joy of Weight Loss program. You'll be fine!

TODAY'S MENU AND ACTIVITY

Keep logging. You're hopefully by now getting the hang of it and it's becoming automatic. You may also, now, begin to see some patterns: eating certain foods every day, at certain times. Eating when emotional. How active or inactive you are. This is all good. Keep working on seeing your patterns by tracking food and activities.

WHAT FOOD/ ACTIVITY	TIME	WHERE	AMOUNTS (in cups)	DOING WHAT (while eating)	FEELINGS (before/after)

PRAYER AND MEDITATION

Take five minutes for silent meditation. Then throughout the day, practice an open-eyed, active meditation. Be on the lookout for how you expect things to be: yourself, others, what you do, and how you feel. Be consciously aware of self-criticisms and judgments. See situations that you're looking forward to, and how they actually end up. Focus on any "entitlement" feelings that may happen. Pay attention to your hopes. Think about how you expected things to be or yourself to be, and that they happened in a totally different way than you ever thought they would. Say to yourself: "I expect(ed) _____ to be _____, and the truth is it is (was) _____."

Day Six

TODAY'S JOYOUS THOUGHT: *Joyous, Conscious Learning*

Once you identify your expectations and begin to see how little they have to do with reality, the way will be more open for you to learn and do new things. It's actually a pleasure to learn and grow, but your mind resists it because of old, destructive habits, useless beliefs, and expectations.

Be aware that you may possibly be holding yourself back, because of these expectations, fears, a residue of self-criticism, or someone or something that hurt you in your past. You may desperately want to lose weight and be healthier. Unconsciously, however, you may feel safer keeping yourself overweight or fat. To learn new ways to shed your "protection pounds" may be threatening to your deep, unconscious psyche. The unconscious psyche may do anything possible to sabotage your efforts. What you need to do, if you suspect there's a part of you that's preventing you from learning and changing, is to become conscious. Learn about your blocks and fears. Consciously accept that they're there, and learn new ways of dealing with them—so you can achieve what you consciously want to do.

Today, in spite of any unconscious desires to remain overweight and out-of-shape, re-read the first four chapters of this book. Keep filling out your food and activity logs.

TODAY'S MENU AND ACTIVITY

You are almost finished with writing a week's worth of food and activity logs. Don't stop now. Make this a very precise, expanded-upon day of recording. You're in the home stretch.

WHAT FOOD/ ACTIVITY	TIME	WHERE	AMOUNTS (in cups)	DOING WHAT (while eating)	FEELINGS (before/after)

PRAYER AND MEDITATION

Take five minutes for silent meditation. Then say this prayer:

"God, please grant me the ability to see how I prevent myself from learning and changing. If it be your will, reveal and illuminate my unconscious limitations. Help me get the power to feel safe to lose weight; help me be the healthier, happy me that I want to be and that I know you want me to be."

Day Seven

TODAY'S JOYOUS THOUGHT: *Allowing Joy and New Experiences*

Today is, as is every day, a continuation. This week, I hope you've praised yourself, made continual commitments, made an effort to read this guide and do it every day, worked on seeing expectations and letting go of them, and are beginning to be aware of how you could be limiting yourself from learning and growing. Be a renegade and a rebel—finish the rest of the book! And make a commitment to continue following this daily guide. You're doing good things for yourself. Congratulations!

Let's take this further, simply, joyously—today. I want you to allow yourself some real joy. I want you to do something really wonderful, positive, and joyous. I want you to finish your food and activity logs and then reward yourself with something that's joyous. Buy yourself some fresh flowers. Take a hot soak-bath, adding some heavenly bath salts or aromatic oils. Don't watch or listen to any negative newscasts or read the newspaper. Go to a concert or on an all-day retreat or conference. Make a drawing or painting or go to a movie or museum with a group of friends or kids.

TODAY'S MENU AND ACTIVITY: *The Big Finish!*

This is it. You're going to do your last day of logging. Be really precise and honest, more than ever today. Go ahead and overeat, be the way you were. Go ahead and make mistakes that you may, by now, know better about. By now you are aware of the food and activity plans. That's OK. Ignore them for today! You have permission!

WHAT FOOD/ ACTIVITY	TIME	WHERE	AMOUNTS (in cups)	DOING WHAT (while eating)	FEELINGS (before/after)

PRAYER AND MEDITATION: *Lighting Your Fire*

Take five minutes for silent meditation. Then, light a candle and stare at the flame. See how it has different parts. Watch it randomly flicker. See how it is dependent on the wax or oil and the wick. It also needs oxygen. It cannot exist without all of these parts.

But what is the fire? No one knows, yet it exists. It's elemental, deeply a part of nature—but we don't know its origins. The fire can warm us with its heat, but it also has the power to destroy us.

Let the candle take you into a deep, peaceful trance.

Once you are very peaceful and transfixed on the flame, feel a similar flame that is burning in you. Feel your inner warmth. See your glow. Know that your flame too is dependent on fuel (food), on a wick (your body), and oxygen (the air you breathe into your lungs from moving). Let your candle warm your being without letting it get out of control and destroying you with too much fuel. Keep the fire of your inner light burning; don't let it go out due to lack of oxygen (from movement).

Now begin to realize that just like the fire of a candle burning bright, your life burns bright. Make sure it has just the right amount of fuel, a healthy body, and enough oxygen.

Day Eight

TODAY'S JOYOUS THOUGHT: *Seeing Patterns*

Congratulations, again, you're on to a new week.

You have a whole week's worth of food and activity data at your service. Now, let's begin a little detective work. We want to discover patterns and connections between your old behaviors and your situations and emotions. We want to make conscious what was once unconscious, unknown, and self-defeating.

DO THIS TODAY: *Connecting Menu and Emotions*

Refer to last week's Daily Companion and pull out a pen or pencil. I want you to draw lines between what foods you ate and the feelings you experienced. Trace connections between difficult feelings and overeating. Line up boredom and eating when you were not hungry. Spot any obvious ties to eating connected to frustrations and/or anxiety. Make connections between feeling happy or satisfied and eating, such as at a celebration or after getting some good news. Do you see any moments when you were lonely and soothed yourself with cake or cookie treats? Were there any times you were feeling lustful or in need of closeness and affection, and instead of getting needs met you stifled the desire with snacks or ice cream? Was there an instance of eating to feel better: to soothe yourself after a long day, or if you felt low-energy and ate candy for a boost? Did you eat snacks or drink a lot of high-caloric drinks because you were shy or embarrassed around others (such as at a social situation, gathering, or party)?

Today, look at only the food and feelings categories. It's enough to see patterns and relationships between emotions and feeding yourself. We'll take more time with the logs and others patterns in the days to come.

TODAY'S MENU

Beginning this week, let's together change the way you eat. We'll do it slowly, starting with breakfast and the morning snack. First, if you have not read Chapter Three, Part II that explains the two Joy of Weight Loss Eating plans, read it now. The main plan, the three meals/three snacks a day is the one which we will begin to use in this first month. The alternate plan, three larger meals, is something you can choose after this initial thirty-day period.

I'd like you to begin following a Joy of Weight Loss Eating Plan, but only for breakfast and the morning snack.

Have a delicious breakfast, one serving each of:

A protein

A grain

A fruit or vegetable

I suggest eating a bowl of cereal, with milk and fruit of your choice.

The grain serving is *one ounce of dry cereal (by weight), or half a cup cooked cereal.* An ounce, in this instance is weight, not volume. Some cereals will tell you how much an ounce is on the label. Some weigh more than others, but you may just estimate if you don't have a scale. Cornflakes don't weigh much, so it's about one cup full; granola weighs a lot, so an ounce is about one-quarter or one-half cup. Other cereals, like wheat or oat squares, or little "O's," would be about three-quarters up to an ounce.

For the protein, have *one cup of milk* in the bowl of cereal.

For fruit, cut up a banana, strawberry, or apple, and put it on top.

To drink, you may have coffee or tea, with a shot of milk in it, and a teaspoon of sugar if you wish.

Don't forget—drink a big glass (eight to ten ounce) of water with your breakfast.

Enjoy a moment of silence before you eat, appreciating all you have and realizing that feeding yourself is serious, important, and joyous. Then, eat slowly, savoring and enjoying each bite.

Make sure to wait twenty minutes after your last bite to feel satisfied. *You will feel that you've had enough.* You may be surprised that so little food can give you enough. This is because you're now eating in balance and proportion. This is "normal" eating at its best.

For the Mid-Morning Snack, two to three hours after breakfast, eat one serving each of:

A grain

A fruit or vegetable (alternated with the last meal)

A protein (alternating meat or dairy, but for only one snack per day)

Drink another big glass of water, after every meal and snack!
Today, let's have pretzels, nuts, and vegetable juice for the snack:

The grain serving is *one ounce pretzels* (about seven small, or two big—refer to the label)

The vegetable is *three-quarters of a cup vegetable juice* (V8, carrot, tomato, mixed, etc.)

The protein is *one-third of a cup* or two tablespoons *peanuts* (or cashews, almonds, etc.)

DRINK: unsweetened iced tea AND a big glass of water (eight to ten ounce). How about club soda?

SILENCE before eating, in gratitude and consciousness

WAIT *at least twenty minutes to feel satisfied.*

For lunch and dinner eat what you like in the amounts you like, and don't feel the need to jump ahead and follow the eating plan for those meals. It's enough to alter only your breakfast and morning snack this week. Take it slow. Please **do not** be overly enthusiastic. Your eating changes should be very, very slow and gradual. Trust me!

TODAY'S ACTIVITY: *A Walk!*

Go for a ten-minute walk today, right after breakfast. It's easy! Just go outside, walk for ten minutes around the block, in a park, or parking lot, or mall. Do it early in the day, if at all possible.

Take five minutes for silent meditation. Then, during your walk, do another open-eye meditation. Walk with your eyes as if newly opened. As you walk, notice any flowers and birds you see. When you do, look closely. Think about them: What colors do they have, what type is it or family does it belong to? Smell a flower, if possible. Follow a bird with your eyes, if possible; see where it goes and its interactions with other birds and with nature.

Then, silently to yourself, thank God for the experience of nature today.

Day Nine

TODAY'S JOYOUS THOUGHT: *Perseverance*

Keep in mind today that your perseverance, your continuation of your self-improvement, will mean the continuation of your life. It's that simple.

The more you resolve to change your habits and lifestyles, using every method available—mind training, nutrition, activity, spiritual surrender, and social bonding—the better you will do.

DO THIS TODAY: *Amounting to Something*

Your education today involves, again, working on seeing patterns in your food logs. This time, I'd like you to study the amount and types of food you ate. Compare your measurements to the USDA Food Guide Pyramid serving sizes on page 45.

1. To the right of each entry, write the approximate number of servings you had of each food item, and put them into one of the five food groups: grain, vegetable, fruit, meat, dairy by marking each item with a "G" "V" "F" "M" or "D."

2. Underline the entry if it contained much fat, salt, or sugar.

3. Now, if the meal or snack was over the suggested number of servings according to the Joy of Weight Loss Eating Plan on pages 42 and 43, circle the entry.

4. Finally, look at the whole day and determine if you got all five food groups in your mouth.

Take a look and see what you've underlined and circled. See where you could use a little improvement in the serving sizes and types of food. This should be a revelation to you, as it is for most people who do this! Feel the joy of accomplishment instead of any guilt or shame that may arise. You've done nothing wrong. Actually, you're totally doing the right thing by becoming *conscious of your past eating habits.*

TODAY'S MENU

Breakfast and the mid-morning snack are on the Joy of Eating Food Plan agenda again today.

Breakfast

MENU	PROTEIN	GRAIN	FRUIT or VEGETABLE
Bagel sandwich, with egg	Two fried or poached eggs	Small bagel (not one of the huge ones, please)	Fruit or vegetable juice of your choice (¾ cup)

- To drink, you may have coffee or tea, with a shot of milk in it, and a teaspoon of sugar if you wish.
- Don't forget—drink a big glass (eight to ten ounce) of water with your breakfast.
- Enjoy a moment of silence before you eat, appreciating all you have and realizing that feeding yourself is serious, important, and joyous. Then, eat slowly, savoring and enjoying each bite.
- Make sure to wait twenty minutes after your last bite to feel satisfied. *You will feel that you've had enough.*

Mid-Morning Snack

Since we had a protein yesterday for the morning snack, let's not have one today.

MENU	PROTEIN	GRAIN	FRUIT or VEGETABLE
Fruit salad, with a caramel-flavored rice cake	None today	A caramel-flavored rice cake	chopped, fresh or canned fruit salad, unsweetened (½ cup)

- DRINK: a big glass (eight to ten ounces) of water, with a squeeze of lemon juice
- SILENCE before eating, in gratitude and consciousness
- WAIT *at least twenty minutes* to feel satisfied.

Today, and this week, only change the breakfast meal and mid-morning snack. Eat whatever and how much you like for lunch, dinner, and snacks. (I'll bet, though, that a little food consciousness is rubbing off on you.) Just be sure not to be overzealous.

TODAY'S ACTIVITY

Walk again for ten minutes today, right after breakfast. Walk to go somewhere or get something. Speed up the walk just a tiny bit. Notice how you feel afterwards, and see if you aren't feeling a little joy because you're moving.

PRAYER AND MEDITATION

Take five minutes for silent meditation. Then, talk with God through this prayer: "God, let me persevere and never give up. Let me not cease trying. If it be your will, grant me the possibility of sticking with my efforts to change until all I've learned and practiced becomes automatic. Amen."

Day Ten

TODAY'S JOYOUS THOUGHT: *Quality Takes Time*

You did not create your weight problem in a short time. It did not take you a week or a month or even one year to put on the extra weight that's bothering you. If you think about it, it took a whole lifetime. Everything you've done up until now has affected the problem: your childhood experiences, adolescence, and adulthood. When you were in your twenties it could have happened, due to social issues, or career, or marriage. Perhaps the weight came on after you turned thirty, or after childbirth. Maybe you are in your forties, fifties, or older, and it's just something that's come time to deal with.

Relax: you have a lifetime to solve the problem. You have lots of time to learn what truly healthy eating means and to get the mental acuity and strength to practice it. Do not give up. Persevere, and you will succeed like never before. Then you'll have the rest of yourself freed-up of weight concerns, to really live your life in a joyous way.

DO THIS TODAY: *A Slow Commitment*

Promise yourself and God that you will commit to taking your time with your weight loss agenda. If you feel the urge to rush, jump the gun, or revert back to your old ways of dieting through deprivation, those old techniques that did you no good, make a new commitment, yet again. Tell yourself: "This takes a lifetime. This is not a diet, not something that'll I'll ever go off. It is a new, normal, and healthy way of life that I'm loving."

Breakfast
A different kind of breakfast might be just the right new thing to get you going today.

M E N U	PROTEIN	GRAIN	FRUIT or VEGETABLE
Swedish breakfast	Piece of smoked salmon (2 to 3 ozs.) or other fish (try whitefish, or pickled herring, or even grilled tuna)	One slice rye bread	Small bowl of ligonberry or apple/blueberry sauce (½ cup)

- To drink, you may have coffee or tea, with a shot of milk in it, and a teaspoon of sugar if you wish.

- Don't forget—drink a big glass (eight to ten ounces) of water with your breakfast.

- Enjoy a moment of silence before you eat, appreciating all you have and realizing that feeding yourself is serious, important, and joyous. Then, eat slowly, savoring and enjoying each bite.

- Make sure to wait twenty minutes after your last bite to feel satisfied. *You will feel that you've had enough.*

Mid-Morning Snack

M E N U	PROTEIN	GRAIN	FRUIT or VEGETABLE
Vegetables with cheese and crackers	Sliced or cubed cheddar, brie, smoked mozzarella, goat, any kind you like (1½ ozs.)	Whole grain or Soda Crackers (5 small)	Mini-carrots or pepper slices—try yellow or red (½ cup, approximately)

- DRINK: a big glass (eight to ten ounces) of seltzer water, with a non-sweetened flavor essence like cherry, orange, or lemon/lime.

- **SILENCE** before eating, in gratitude and consciousness

- **WAIT** at least twenty minutes to feel satisfied.

TODAY'S ACTIVITY

Another walk would be nice. Ten minutes is all you need. If it's raining, walk inside a shopping center or mall or around the office hallway.

PRAYER AND MEDITATION

Slow down! I mean *really* slow down and take your time. Sit for ten minutes in quiet meditation next to a stream or brook. Close your eyes and listen to the gentle water endlessly flowing by, giving you an unequalled feeling of liquid tranquility. If you can't get to a source of water today, sit and listen to tranquil music or a tape of the sea or a river.

Just before you're done, say this prayer: "God, please help me take my time. Help me not to rush. Help me to know that I have enough time and that everything will be all right, in good time. Amen."

Day Eleven

TODAY'S JOYOUS THOUGHT: *Do Something Different*

Since every day is a new day, with different happenings, changing weather, work needs, and people needs, you might as well acknowledge the difference. You might as well do something new, to help yourself become new!

What could you do that's new? How about something physical? That would be good for both your body and mind.

DO THIS TODAY

Here are some ideas of new things: swing on a swing, kick a ball around, go swimming, walk to the store and back, play wall-ball, borrow a dog and walk it (or add extra walk time, or go somewhere new if you already have a dog). Go to a new park. There are lots of things to do. Think of something and just do it. Once you've started, you'll get into it and have fun, I promise!

Breakfast

This morning, have an "s" treat! Eat things that start with the letter "S": sausage (veggie), scones, strawberries!

M E N U	PROTEIN	GRAIN	FRUIT or VEGETABLE
"S"	Veggie sausage (two ounces, one patty or two links)	Small scone (about the size of a slice of bread)	A bowl of strawberries (½ cup)

- To drink, you may have coffee or tea, with a shot of milk in it, and a teaspoon of sugar if you wish.

- Don't forget—drink a big glass (eight to ten ounce) of water with your breakfast.

- Enjoy a moment of silence before you eat, appreciating all you have and realizing that feeding yourself is serious, important, and joyous. Then, eat slowly, savoring and enjoying each bite.

- Make sure to wait twenty minutes after your last bite to feel satisfied. *You will feel that you've had enough.*

Mid-Morning Snack

Since you had protein yesterday for the morning snack, try not having it today.

M E N U	PROTEIN	GRAIN	FRUIT or VEGETABLE
	None right now	Pretzel nuggets (½ cup)	Apple-cranberry juice (¾ cup)

- DRINK: One large (eight to ten ounce) glass of water.

TODAY'S ACTIVITY

If you can, do one of the new and different activities that I suggested to you, above. If not, then *at least walk for ten minutes again today.* Pick up the pace a little more, and really enjoy yourself!

PRAYER AND MEDITATION

Do something different with your meditation today, too. Make it a reflection.

In a quiet place of solitude, close your eyes, take ten deep breaths and then think about the different thing you did today and how it made you feel. Think on how joyous it was to do something different and new. Reflect on the idea of change, how it is inevitable and unavoidable, and how much easier your life would be if you could just change easily without resistance. Contemplate how you have made your life harder in the past by not changing and resisting the natural flow of life. If you feel sad or sorry about how you've blocked yourself, congratulations! Go ahead and allow yourself a little sadness for a moment. Then move on, let go of it, and say this prayer to yourself and to God: "Dear Spirit of Change, dear God within me, allow me to not get in the way of change. If it be thy will, let me be an open book for you to write my new life story in. Let me go with your flow and not get in the way. I'm beginning to love you, God. Let me begin to love myself in you, too. Amen."

Then take five more minutes for silent meditation.

Day Twelve

TODAY'S JOYOUS THOUGHT: *Loving the Hate*

Today is a very special day in this program. Today, I encourage you to do something with the blocks and self-hatred deep inside you that are holding you back. They are there, although you may be unaware of their presence. They are there as evidenced by your overweight condition, there when you self-criticize or put yourself down in public or private, there when you feel afraid of doing things that are really not so difficult. You may expect me to tell you to get rid of them. You may be surprised when I don't!

I encourage you not only to face your blocks, fears, and self-hatred and admit they are there inside you, but I suggest you let them exist!

DO THIS TODAY

Today, please make sure to do two things that are special and vitally important for your complete and joyous weight loss. Do not let your internal saboteur prevent you or convince you to procrastinate! (And it will try, due to its own desire for self-preservation.)

1. Confide to yourself and to God that you have some self-hate, fears, blocks, and problems that have been holding you back from changing and being your best. Go ahead and do it now. Say a prayer: "OK, I have some problems, and I'm having a hard time dealing with them myself." (Know that it is OK to have problems and self-hate.)

2. Think of a trustworthy friend, trusted spiritual counselor or therapist, or anonymous meeting fellowship to whom you can confide your problems and self-hatred. Make an appointment or plan to get together to talk with this person or go to a meeting tomorrow.

TODAY'S MENU

Breakfast

MENU	PROTEIN	GRAIN	FRUIT or VEGETABLE
A bowl of cereal	Milk (1 cup)	Cereal (1 oz.)	Banana, apples, or berries (½ cup)

- To drink, you may have coffee or tea, with a shot of milk in it, and a teaspoon of sugar if you wish.
- Don't forget—drink a big glass (eight to ten ounce) of water with your breakfast.
- Enjoy a moment of silence before you eat, appreciating all you have and realizing that feeding yourself is serious, important, and joyous. Then, eat slowly, savoring and enjoying each bite.
- Make sure to wait twenty minutes after your last bite to feel satisfied. You will feel that you've had enough.

Mid-Morning Snack

How about some protein today with the snack, since you didn't have any yesterday?

MENU	PROTEIN	GRAIN	FRUIT or VEGETABLE
	Peanuts (⅓ cup, or 2 tbs approx., not buttered)	Popcorn (1 cup)	Apple juice (¾ cup)

- DRINK: One large (eight to ten ounce) glass of water.

TODAY'S ACTIVITY

Walk ten minutes today or do something new and fun! (See Chapter Three, Part II for some ideas.) Make sure to do it early in the day, so you do not put it off.

Take five minutes for silent meditation. Then pray: "God, as I prepare myself for you, let me become aware of my shortcomings, blocks, self-hatred, self-criticism, and self-caused problems. Give me the power to see them, acknowledge them, and begin to live more easily with them. I know I can't keep making things hard on myself. I know I'm my own worst enemy. Help me to love myself more and begin even to love that side of me that is hardest to love."

Day Thirteen ⸾

TODAY'S JOYOUS THOUGHT: *Letting Go of the Problems*

This is a joyous day of celebration! Instead of thinking that what you're going to do today is hard, embarrassing, or shameful, think of it as joyously liberating! Today, you're going to release your self-imposed imprisonment of self-hate, emotional misery, blocks, fears, and shame. You're going to tell someone that your life is hard, and that you have problems.

Chances are, they'll commiserate and tell you their problems, too!

DO THIS TODAY

I hope you made an appointment to get together with someone you can confide in. If so, then, when you meet, just get into a light and easy conversation with small talk. Ask this other person about their life, and listen. Keep talking. At just the right moment, when they're listening to you, share a problem that you're having, and say: "You know, life is just really hard, and I've come to realize that I make it hard on myself. I've also come to know that I just can't do everything myself. I just cannot do it all alone! I guess we all need help, don't we? I sure do!"

Bingo! There you will have done it. Simple! Just weave into conversation these vital truths about yourself (in your own words):

1. "Life is difficult, and I have problems."

2. "I am holding myself back because of old habits, self-hate, fears, and emotional blocks."

3. "I need help. I cannot do everything myself."

Once this is done, be sure to celebrate your personal liberation. Have a joyous and delightful moment, because you've let go of your problems by confiding them to someone else.

(If you didn't make an appointment, and you are still holding back, there are several other ways to do this essential work.) Try:

- Getting into a conversation with a complete stranger who doesn't know you and you may never see again.
- Going to a meeting at a place of worship or health center.
- Calling Overeaters Anonymous and going to one of their meetings.
- Calling an anonymous "listening line" service.

TODAY'S MENU

Breakfast

MENU	PROTEIN	GRAIN	FRUIT or VEGETABLE
Strawberry Yogurt Banana Split	Yogurt (½ cup) almonds, chopped, toasted (⅓ cup)	Vanilla wafers (four approx.)	Banana (½) Strawberries (¼ cup)

DRINK: **One large (eight to ten ounce) glass of water.**

Mid-Morning Snack

Today is a no-protein snack day.

MENU	PROTEIN	GRAIN	FRUIT or VEGETABLE
		Small muffin	Fruit cup (½ cup)

DRINK: **One large (eight to ten ounce) glass of water.**

TODAY'S ACTIVITY

Why not walk with your friend for ten minutes? However, walk for at least ten minutes today. Pick up the pace a little bit, too.

PRAYER AND MEDITATION

As you go through your day today, open your heart and eyes and see how you are making yourself miserable, often creating your own problems. Notice how you try to solve everything yourself and how futile it is. See how you really need help. Pray: "God, let me not only see my own problems, but show me the way to confide them to others, admitting I have been holding myself back and that I need help. Amen."

Be sure to take five minutes for silent meditation, some time during our day, today.

Day Fourteen

TODAY'S JOYOUS THOUGHT: *Surrender*

Today is the most important day of your life. This is the day you give your life to God. This is the moment when you surrender all of your problems. Do not wait, whatever you do. Put your faith into action today and do not delay one second longer. It's actually a simple act and takes only a few minutes.

DO THIS TODAY

Go to page 33, the "Take Joy in Surrendering" section in Chapter Three, Part I. Follow the instructions you find there. Now is the time to actually do this. You will find it to be the single most liberating, most powerful, and most beautiful and joyous thing you've ever done. Do not hold back. Save your life and unite with God this moment.

TODAY'S MENU

Breakfast

MENU	PROTEIN	GRAIN	FRUIT or VEGETABLE
Hot oatmeal	Milk (I cup)	Cooked oatmeal (½ cup)	Raisins (¼ cup)

- **DRINK: One large (eight to ten ounce) glass of water.**

Mid-Morning Snack

MENU	PROTEIN	GRAIN	FRUIT or VEGETABLE
	Toasted soybeans (½ cup)	Pretzels (7 small, 2 big)	Cherry tomatoes (½ cup)

- **DRINK: One large (eight to ten ounce) glass of water.**

TODAY'S ACTIVITY

Walk ten minutes at the end of the day. With each step, thank God for your life.

PRAYER AND MEDITATION

Take five minutes for silent meditation, and then time for a prayer.

There is only one prayer that I ever pray. I think this is the only one you will ever truly need, too: "God, I need help. Show me Your way, and give me the power to do Your will."

Day Fifteen

TODAY'S JOYOUS THOUGHT: *Sweet Release*

Be joyous, because you have help. You are not alone anymore. God is there, always, helping you. He will be there in all ways. All you need to do is ask. Feel free to ask God for help. Rejoice in your freedom of knowledge that it's not all up to you to do everything alone anymore. You do not have to achieve the impossible or be perfect any longer. You don't have to always feel impotent, small, and powerless.

Rejoice that you have completed the second week. You have accomplished a lot!

DO THIS TODAY

Completely allow yourself to feel the sweet release of your life to God. You have done the one most important thing a human being could ever do. You are now joyously more successful than you know. Rest assured you will be absolutely fine, no matter what may come, because you have empowered yourself with God, due to the Grace of God!

TODAY'S MENU

Beginning this week, we'll add lunch and the afternoon snack on your Joy of Weight Loss Eating Plan. Again, you may vary the suggested foods you eat, as long as you keep to the structured plan. I offer you menu suggestions simply as a helpful guide and to teach you moderation and healthy, joyous eating.

Breakfast

M E N U	PROTEIN	GRAIN	FRUIT or VEGETABLE
A bowl of cereal	Milk (I cup)	Cereal (I oz., about ¾ cup average)	Banana (I, cut-up)

To drink, you may have coffee or tea, with a shot of milk in it, and a teaspoon of sugar if you wish.

- **Don't forget—drink a big glass (eight to ten ounce) of water with your breakfast.**

- **Enjoy a moment of silence before you eat, appreciating all you have and realizing that feeding yourself is serious, important, and joyous. Then, eat slowly, savoring and enjoying each bite.**

- **Make sure to wait twenty minutes after your last bite to feel satisfied. You will feel that you've had enough.**

Mid-Morning Snack

As you had a protein in the snack yesterday, skip it today. We can give it to you this afternoon, besides!

M E N U	PROTEIN	GRAIN	FRUIT or VEGETABLE
		Bread (I slice)	Fruit spread, unsweetened. Try raspberry or apricot!. (2 tbs)

DRINK: **One large (eight to ten ounce) glass of water.**

Lunch

Just like every meal and snack, lunch consists of one serving each of:

- **A protein (meat or dairy group, alternating)**

- **A grain**

- **A fruit or vegetable (alternating each meal and snack)**

We want you to eat from all five food groups the minimum number of servings each day. If you have not read Chapter Three, Part II about The Joy of Weight Loss Eating Plan and the USDA Food Guide Pyramid, please do it!

M E N U	PROTEIN	GRAIN	FRUIT or VEGETABLE
Sandwich: grilled chicken	Grilled chicken (2 ozs.)	Small bun	Lettuce and tomato, pickles on the side

- DRINK: **One large (eight to ten ounce) glass of water.**

Afternoon Snack

For the afternoon snack, have another grain and fruit or vegetable—alternating the fruit or vegetable. Since you had a vegetable with lunch, have a fruit for this snack. Also, one snack per day should have protein. Since you didn't have protein for the mid-morning snack, have some protein this afternoon. You should have the afternoon snack two to three hours after you finished lunch, so you won't get hungry as the day goes on.

M E N U	PROTEIN	GRAIN	FRUIT or VEGETABLE
Gourmet cheese, crackers and fruit	Brie cheese (1½ oz. natural)	Oat-bran crackers (5, average)	Kiwi fruit (medium)

- DRINK: **One large (eight to ten ounce) glass of water.**

TODAY'S ACTIVITY

As we are now adding structured eating, we are also adding a little more to your daily active, physical movement. This week, beginning today, you need to be active for twenty minutes. This could be a twenty-minute walk or any other activity you choose. Refer to the Joy of Weight Loss Activity Plan section on pages 68 and 69 of Chapter Three, Part II. Do something different!

Most importantly, make it *enjoyable.*

PRAYER AND MEDITATION

Take five minutes for silent meditation. Be thankful to God, today, for your life, your spiritual surrender, and your freedom.

TODAY'S JOYOUS THOUGHT: *Joyous Eating*

You are now exactly two/thirds on The Joy of Weight Loss Eating Plan. You are slowly but surely altering your eating habits and consumption lifestyle.

Be sure to pick foods you enjoy—foods that you like to eat, are hungry for, and that are delicious and satisfying.

If you eat a little too much, don't worry. Just eat a little less the next time. Or you can always skip a snack or meal (but only one, please). Skipping more than one meal or snack time will make you ravenous, which may make you eat much too much the next time. The idea is to eat small meals and snacks throughout the day (every two to three hours maximum) so you will never get too hungry. Also, if you want more at a meal, go ahead and have two servings but then eliminate the in-between snack.

DO THIS TODAY

As you eat each bite of food today, chew it thoroughly (at least ten times). Enjoy the flavor, texture, aroma, quality, and sensation of the food. Be thankful that you have enough to eat when so many people in the world do not. Be conscious of eating; make it a joyous occasion every time.

TODAY'S MENU

Breakfast

M E N U	PROTEIN	GRAIN	FRUIT or VEGETABLE
Fruit yogurt and toast	Yogurt (I cup)	Slice of toast	Chopped pineapple (½ cup)

- To drink, you may have coffee or tea, with a shot of milk in it, and a teaspoon of sugar if you wish.

- Don't forget—drink a big glass (eight to ten ounce) of water with your breakfast.

- Enjoy a moment of silence before you eat, appreciating all you have and realizing that feeding yourself is serious, important, and joyous. Then, eat slowly, savoring and enjoying each bite.

- Make sure to wait twenty minutes after your last bite to feel satisfied. You will feel that you've had enough.

Mid-Morning Snack

MENU	PROTEIN	GRAIN	FRUIT or VEGETABLE
	Chicken leg (one average size)	Biscuit	Coleslaw with vinegar dressing (½ cup)

- Don't forget—drink a big glass (eight to ten ounce) of water.

- Enjoy a moment of silence before you eat, appreciating all you have and realizing that feeding yourself is serious, important, and joyous. Then, eat slowly, savoring and enjoying each bite.

- Make sure to wait twenty minutes after your last bite to feel satisfied. You will feel that you've had enough.

Lunch

MENU	PROTEIN	GRAIN	FRUIT or VEGETABLE
Salad: nicoise	Anchovies or tuna fish (2 ozs.)	Croutons (1 oz. or ½ cup)	Raw spinach and lettuce (½ cup), potatoes, tomatoes (¼ cup)

- DRINK: One large (eight to ten ounce) glass of water.

Afternoon Snack

MENU	PROTEIN	GRAIN	FRUIT or VEGETABLE
	None right now	Pretzel nuggets (10)	Apple-cranberry juice (¾ cup)

- DRINK: One large (eight to ten ounce) glass of water.

TODAY'S ACTIVITY

Another twenty-minute jaunt, dance session, swim, stretch or yoga class. Do it! Don't delay!

PRAYER AND MEDITATION

Take five minutes for silent meditation.

Before every meal, during every bite, say: "Thank you, God."

TODAY'S JOYOUS THOUGHT: *Enough*

When you're feeling emotionally empty, there's never enough. You need more comfort, pleasure, soothing, affection, and food. Thank God you now have God in your life. Thank God you've had enough of your weight problems and have asked for help and are receiving it. Now you don't need to feel that deep emptiness anymore.

With spiritual food, you always have enough. You are filled with Divine Joy. It's a far greater feeling of satisfaction than you get from a lot of food. You feel emotionally complete, because you know you're not alone. Now there's a purpose to your life.

Now you're learning what healthy, moderate eating is. You're eating a lot less than you used to and you are now hopefully feeling satisfied sooner and in a more complete, balanced way. You don't need as much food any longer because your whole life is more satisfying, balanced, and complete.

DO THIS TODAY

When you finish each meal or snack, wait for twenty minutes. This lets your body tell your brain you've eaten.

If you have a problem stopping after you have eaten your portions, ask God for help. Ask Him to give you stopping power. Train your mind and be still. Let the nagging temptation float away, into God's hands. Then leave the food; get up from the table and do something else. The temptation will go away in about five minutes or so. Practicing this, time and time again, will eventually give you complete freedom from overeating. You will have given your habits a rest and your body time to get used to being treated with care and affection—something you've been truly hungry for for a long time.

TODAY'S MENU

Breakfast

MENU	PROTEIN	GRAIN	FRUIT or VEGETABLE
A bowl of cereal	Milk (1 cup)	Cereal (1 oz., about ¾ cup average)	Fruit, sliced (½ cup)

- **DRINK: One large (eight to ten ounce) glass of water.**

Mid-Morning Snack

MENU	PROTEIN	GRAIN	FRUIT or VEGETABLE
	Bouillon (1 cup)	Roll	Applesauce (½ cup)

- **DRINK: One large (eight to ten ounce) glass of water.**

Lunch

MENU	PROTEIN	GRAIN	FRUIT or VEGETABLE
Sandwich: tuna salad	Tuna salad (2 ozs)	Small roll	Lettuce and tomato, pickles and carrot sticks on the side

- **DRINK: One large (eight to ten ounce) glass of water.**

Afternoon Snack

MENU	PROTEIN	GRAIN	FRUIT or VEGETABLE
	None (had it this morning)	2 flavored rice or popcorn cakes	Banana

- **DRINK: One large (eight to ten ounce) glass of water.**

TODAY'S ACTIVITY

Another twenty-minute walk. Go and pick up the dry-cleaning on foot. Or shop for a new watch, so you can time your activities! Just walk to the jewelry or department store.

PRAYER AND MEDITATION

Go to your private sanctuary, where you can be alone with God. Turn off the lights and shut the door. Sit comfortably and close your eyes. Imagine yourself walking through a beautiful forest—deep into the woods, down a path filled with ferns, trees, ivy, birds singing, flowers blooming, rays of sunlight cascading down. Take five deep cleansing breaths. Continue going down the path. You come to a little clearing. There, in the woods, you see an object. Imagine that the object means something symbolically important to you. Mentally pick it up. Hold it, feel it, smell it, caress it. Let yourself have the feeling that the object is speaking to you—not in words, but still meaningfully. Let it say: "There is enough. You are enough." Know that the object is a gift from God, especially for you. Put the object in your pocket and turn and walk back down the forest path, back through the woods, back to your private sanctuary. Now take a deep breath and open your eyes. Know that your important, meaningful object is symbolically in your pocket, with you always. You will always have it and you will always have enough.

Day Eighteen

TODAY'S JOYOUS THOUGHT: *Feeling Alive*

In yesterday's meditation, you picked an object that was meaningful and important to you as a symbol that you have enough. Today, let's pick some real symbols that demonstrate and remind you that you are alive and well, a part of nature, and that you not only are enough and have enough but that you are blessed with joyous abundance.

DO THIS TODAY

Surround yourself with symbols of life. Pick some fresh flowers and place in a simple but nice vase or cup. Watch their cycle of life: opening, blooming, and then wilting. Get an inexpensive houseplant and care for it every day, giving it enough water and light, but not too much! A little tree or bush in a pot, or a bonsai might be really refreshing in the house. Or how about an animal or fish? Dogs really are our best friends; or a cat is nice to stroke and pet. A bowl of goldfish could brighten your life and give you endless hours of pleasure. Of course, caring for animals is a great responsibility, one that you cannot enter into lightly. If you choose to adopt a pet, make the commitment to give it the utmost care and love possible. It's different than getting a houseplant!

If the above seems like too much to take care of right now, how about buying a really beautiful picture or poster of a photograph or work of art that gives you the feeling of being alive? It could be anything that touches your soul and reminds you, too, that you are alive and a part of nature.

Breakfast

M E N U	PROTEIN	GRAIN	FRUIT or VEGETABLE
Western egg/ muffin sandwich	2 eggs, scrambled	English muffin	Cut-up onion, pepper, mushroom (½ cup)

- To drink, you may have coffee or tea, with a shot of milk in it, and a teaspoon of sugar if you wish.

- Don't forget—drink a big glass (eight to ten ounce) of water with your breakfast.

- Enjoy a moment of silence before you eat, appreciating all you have and realizing that feeding yourself is serious, important, and joyous. Then, eat slowly, savoring and enjoying each bite.

- Make sure to wait twenty minutes after your last bite to feel satisfied. You will feel that you've had enough.

Mid-Morning Snack

M E N U	PROTEIN	GRAIN	FRUIT or VEGETABLE
Three-bean salad	Chickpeas and kidney beans in the salad (1 cup)	Flat bread (two sticks)	Three-bean salad (½ cup vegetables). The third been is a green bean!

- DRINK: One large (eight to ten ounce) glass of water.

Lunch

M E N U	PROTEIN	GRAIN	FRUIT or VEGETABLE
Sandwich: Tuna salad	Tuna salad (2 ozs.)	Small roll	Lettuce and tomato, pickles and carrot sticks on the side

DRINK: One large (eight to ten ounce) glass of water.

Afternoon Snack

Since you had protein for the morning snack, you need not have it again this afternoon.

M E N U	PROTEIN	GRAIN	FRUIT or VEGETABLE
		Popcorn, (1 cup, approx., unbuttered)	Fruit juice, try peach nectar, or guava! (¾ cup)

- DRINK: **One large (eight to ten ounce) glass of water.**

TODAY'S ACTIVITY

Move joyously for twenty minutes today. How about signing up for a class at a nearby recreation center or making an appointment with a personal trainer or coach? A yoga or stretch class is a wonderful mini-vacation while a rousing beginning hip-hop class is awesome!

PRAYER AND MEDITATION

Sit quietly, first thing in the morning, right after your shower or bath and before breakfast. Be in a private room, with no noise or distractions. Sit on the floor, on a cushion or mat, legs crossed. (If you cannot do this, a straight-back chair is fine.)

Close your eyes. Let your mind travel. Picture yourself on a magic glider flying up and up through the clouds, up to space, beyond the planets, and into the stars. You are moving further away from earth and all of your cares and worries. Now you are in far-outer space and it is quiet, marvelously still, totally peaceful, and remote. Slowly, your glider/space vehicle dissolves away and you are floating limitless, in the hands of the Universe. You are safe, sound, comfortable, alive, and well.

You are there, quiet and alone, except for one thing that is there, deeper inside you than you. A part of you is witnessing and watching, present and attentive. Can you feel that part? It doesn't talk in words, but it's behind your words. You cannot see it, but you feel it's seeing through you. It is something you cannot quite feel with your small human senses, but it is there—present and strong. You feel it with a different, new sense in you. It is warm, serene, strong, and big. Not only is this presence in you, it is also surrounding you. It is at once as vast as everything in the 100 billion galaxies we know of and as vast as the infinite numbers of galaxies we do not. It is as small as the hundreds of trillions of quarks in the atoms that make you who you are. This presence is alive and real. You know it is there with everything you know, with everything that is you, and is everything in this creation. This presence is God. Because there is no other way to describe it in these limited words and concepts, it is best to experience it, to let the Reality that is you reveal its Godliness to you. It will. Just ask. It will answer because it is a part of you. You are alive because it created you.

Take ten deep breaths and go into God's presence. Let your entire being focus on God. Now take ten more deep breaths, as you travel down through the stars and planets, back through the clouds, and slowly, softly back to earth. You return, back through the roof of your house, effortlessly landing in your sanctuary, safe and sound. The difference this time, however, is that you've brought back your realization that God is there, with you. Open your eyes, see the world and your life fully alive and new again, today.

Day Nineteen ⤺

TODAY'S JOYOUS THOUGHT: *Symbols of God*

The last two days you've been thinking of symbols and visualizing what's important and meaningful. You've gathered items that convey beautiful things in your life. Living things, plants, an animal, photographs, keepsakes—anything that is special.

Today, think about important symbols in another way. Think about how God shows Himself to you, as symbols of His love and care. Perhaps it's in a beautiful sunset, or a flower, or a song on the radio, or a feeling or intuition, a miraculous healing you've received, or passages from the Bible, or spiritual text that stood out.

Truth is, we are God's creations, living symbols of His brilliance and creativity. So are others, so is nature, so is everything we do. We are His created and gathered symbols.

Therefore, be sure to live your life well, because you, yourself, are a symbol of God. Take excellent care of yourself, and do your best in everything you do.

DO THIS TODAY

Make a little altar or shrine in your sanctuary or special place. Just get a little table, or simply a box, and put a nice cloth over it. Make it beautiful and special, in your own symbolic way.

Gather together the symbols you've chosen the last two days and place them neatly on your altar. Carefully place pictures of important people whom you love, or pictures of beautiful nature scenes, or a special flower or plant, and other objects that mean something dear to you. Perhaps it's a bell or candle or a special piece of jewelry or work of art that speaks your heart and soul, of your love for God and His creation.

Let this altar be a special place, a point of honor, a sacred spot in your life. Every time you see it, let it remind you that things are different for you in your life, because you love God and are thankful for all you have—good and bad, sorrowful or joyful— and of your desires to change for the better, one day at a time.

Just one more thing: don't let the altar or what's on it become your focus of worship to God. Go directly to Him in prayer, deep inside you. There's no substitute for a direct and complete personal relationship with our Divine Creator, and there's no symbol on earth (or even in the Universe) that can replace God Himself. Remember, the altar and everything on it are only *symbols*.

TODAY'S MENU

MENU	PROTEIN	GRAIN	FRUIT or VEGETABLE
Breakfast on the run: muffin, fruit yogurt	Yogurt (1 cup)	Carrot or bran muffin (small size)	Cut-up fresh fruit, apples, banana, cherries, mixed into the yogurt (½ cup)

- To drink, you may have coffee or tea, with a shot of milk in it, and a teaspoon of sugar if you wish.

- Don't forget—drink a big glass (eight to ten ounce) of water with your breakfast.

- Enjoy a moment of silence before you eat, appreciating all you have and realizing that feeding yourself is serious, important and joyous. Then, eat slowly, savoring and enjoying each bite.

- Make sure to wait twenty minutes after your last bite to feel satisfied. You will feel that you've had enough.

Mid-Morning Snack

MENU	PROTEIN	GRAIN	FRUIT or VEGETABLE
Juice and cookies	Skip it this morning	Cookies (2 small whole grain, preferably, fruit juice sweetened, if possible)	Fruit juice. If you like, mix it with club soda or seltzer ($^3/_4$ cup)

- **DRINK:** One large (eight to ten ounce) glass of water.

Lunch

MENU	PROTEIN	GRAIN	FRUIT or VEGETABLE
Pizza with veggies	Shredded cheese ($1^1/_2$ ozs.)	Crust (1 slice)	Tomato sauce. Onions, green pepper, broccoli, tomatoes ($^1/_2$ cup)

- **DRINK:** One large (eight to ten ounce) glass of water.

Afternoon Snack

Since you didn't have protein for the morning snack, you should have it this afternoon.

MENU	PROTEIN	GRAIN	FRUIT or VEGETABLE
	Cheese (2 slices processed or $1^1/_2$ ozs. natural)	Whole wheat crackers (about 6)	Carrots and celery

- **DRINK:** One large (eight to ten ounce glass of water.)

TODAY'S ACTIVITY

Move joyously for twenty minutes today. How about going to a playground and swinging on a swing like you used to do?

PRAYER & MEDITATION

"God, I want to see you in myself, in everything I do and say, and in all I see and do. I ask you to show yourself to me, in ways that I am able to sense your divine presence. I love you a lot, God, and I know you love me. Amen."

Day Twenty

TODAY'S JOYOUS THOUGHT: *Counting Your Blessings*

How marvelous you are! You're alive and well, doing your thing, doing your best. Not only are you alive, you're becoming aware of being alive. You are becoming more and more conscious of life and your importance in it, every day. You're letting yourself be, in the way that you are, and not being so upset over it. At least, I hope you are!

As a way to expand your consciousness and not be upset over the little things in life, it's most helpful to count your blessings. It's also a terrific survival mechanism that you can employ whenever you are in trouble, feeling down, blue, or suffering. Seeing what's good in your life, instead of focusing on what's not, will instantly snap you back to reality and help you cope with your challenges and make the most of the many opportunities that God has given you.

I'm not saying to avoid pain and sorrow, I'm just suggesting that there's always another side to consider. If you want to experience a range of emotions, making a list will help you regain balance.

DO THIS TODAY

Get out a piece of paper and make a list of ten things you are blessed with in your life: little things, big things, seemingly irrelevant things that actually are not so. You must do this today, even though you may well be trying to talk yourself out of it this very moment. Just begin the list now. Start with reading this book: Hold it in your hand, think about it, put hope and action into your life. This is very positive. It is in itself a blessing that you're allowing and that God has given you. Number two: Give thanks you're alive and able to read at all. You are still breathing! Number three: Think of something nice you're wearing. Number four: Look around you. Whether you're in a room or outside, you're blessed with a place to be right now. Number five: You have things to do, finish, and accomplish—in other words, you have opportunities. There you are. There's half the list. Now think of five more things you're lucky to have. Those could be a home, a job, a family, a place of worship, food to eat, transportation, a bed, the ability to think and reason, and on and on. Make a list and love it! Count your blessings and allow yourself some joy in having them!

Breakfast

How about something really different for breakfast? A European-style beginning.

MENU	PROTEIN	GRAIN	FRUIT or VEGETABLE
	Sliced assorted cheeses (2 slices)	Rye flat bread (1 slice)	Olives, pickles, radish

- To drink, you may have coffee or tea, with a shot of milk in it, and a teaspoon of sugar if you wish.

- Don't forget—drink a big glass (eight to ten ounce) of water with your breakfast.

- Enjoy a moment of silence before you eat, appreciating all you have and realizing that feeding yourself is serious, important, and joyous. Then, eat slowly, savoring and enjoying each bite.

- Make sure to wait twenty minutes after your last bite to feel satisfied. You will feel that you've had enough.

Mid-Morning Snack

Just to remind you, we're varying protein between afternoon and lunch, and vegetable and fruits between breakfast and lunch. Since you had protein yesterday afternoon, skip it this morning, and since you had vegetables for breakfast (novel idea, right?!) have some fruit now.

MENU	PROTEIN	GRAIN	FRUIT or VEGETABLE
Smoothie and cookies		Two small cookies of your choice (try to have healthy ones, sweetened with fruit sugar, if possible)	A small smoothie consisting of apple juice (¼ cup), banana (½), a couple of strawberries (½ cup) herb-fruit iced tea and crushed ice (½ cup), in a blender

- DRINK: One large (eight to ten ounce) glass of water.

Lunch

MENU	PROTEIN	GRAIN	FRUIT or VEGETABLE
Salad: tossed	Shredded cheese (1½ oz.)	Croutons (1 oz. or ½ cup)	Raw spinach and lettuce (¼ cup), tomatoes, celery (¼ cup)

- DRINK: One large (eight to ten ounce) glass of water.

Afternoon Snack

M E N U	PROTEIN	GRAIN	FRUIT or VEGETABLE
Chinese Dim Sum (dumplings)	Pork filling in the Dim Sum (2 to 3 ozs.)	Three Dim sum (dumpling dough)	Lychees (½ cup)

- **DRINK: One large (eight to ten ounce) glass of water.**

TODAY'S ACTIVITY

Twenty minutes of joyous movement is yours today. If it's raining, stay inside and do a "building romp." This is fun and a little wild. The only requirement is a building with about ten floors and access to the stairs and hallways.

Walk up one flight of stairs. Walk around the hallway, slowly. Walk another flight up. Walk around the third floor hallway a little faster. Now begin whistling a happy tune from the movie "Mary Poppins!" Walk up the next flight of stairs. Pay no attention to others around you, except to laugh with them, and get them to join you! Walk around the fourth floor hallway at a slightly faster pace. Then go up the stairs, around, up, around, up... to where you've walked fifteen minutes. Stop for thirty seconds, catch your breath, and then walk down the stairs, slowly for the last five minutes until you reach your starting point. Be sure to wear a smile on your face! It's a little silly, but it makes you feel *great*! Try it.

PRAYER AND MEDITATION

Take five minutes for silent meditation. Then, share your gratitude and joy!

Pray: "God, thank you for all that I have. All of the many blessings: the ones that I am aware of and especially the ones that I'm not. And, God, thank you even for the blessings in disguise—the things I think are problems and sorrows. The more I live my life I discover that you were always there, guiding me rightly and helping me learn and grow by living my life in a joyously active way. Amen."

TODAY'S JOYOUS THOUGHT: *The Joy of Commitment*

I was talking with a very close friend recently, talking about God, and how I thought all religions and spiritual paths were important and all led to the same God. She said she agreed, but she tickled me with joy when she said that it was like going to a train station. "All of those trains may bring you to the station, to the big city," she said. "But you've got to pick one train and get on board! If you don't, you don't go anywhere!"

Boy, did that ring a bell! You gotta get on the train! Like the New York Lottery slogan says: "You gotta be in it to win it!" You have to make a commitment and ride it out until you get to where you want to go.

The same is true with weight loss. You have to commit to changing your lifestyle and habits in order to see any progress. Just sitting, continuing to overeat, not moving—saying to yourself that you'll start tomorrow or you'll go on a diet right after that triple-fudge, brownie-delight, pecan-encrusted, whipped-cream-topped cherry-ized mountain of fat—won't do anything except get you fatter and more miserable.

Most folks who want to lose weight are so jaded and tired of huge, everything-at-once dieting that they can't begin to start again. The answer, therefore, is to make a lot of little starts, a lot of little commitments, all day, every day. Commit to having a banana instead of a brownie. Commit to having one helping, not three. Commit to walking twenty minutes a day, instead of an intense ninety-minute advanced aerobics class once every six months. Commit to asking for help from God again today and taking it slowly in little increments, instead of trying to change everything all at once by yourself again.

The Joy of Weight Loss Contract

I promise and commit to God and myself to follow The Joy of Weight Loss Plans today, all day, to the best of my ability.

I will allow joy into my life. I will not hold back emotions. I will be myself, as real as I can be.

I further commit that if I have a problem, I will ask for help. I will then allow myself to get over it.

I surrender my problems to God as I understand Him, and put my life under His care and direction.

I will not diet or deprive myself. I will eat small servings from all food groups in balance, and I will be active today.

I will endeavor to see God in others, be a good listener, and help other people in need if I can.

If I make a mistake, I will just admit it, ask for help and forgiveness, and then get over it and move on.

Most importantly, I will know that I am very valuable, I am not alone, and I will allow joy into my life.

    In Gratitude,
    I commit for today,

_____

(signature)   *(date)*

DO THIS TODAY

Every hour, make a little commitment to stay with this program—at least one, better yet many. Commit to making a commitment. Commit to eating exactly the one serving of three food groups for your next meal or snack. Commit to getting outside and moving for twenty minutes as soon as possible.

If you do it little by little, one commitment at a time, one day at a time, then it suddenly becomes not only manageable, but joyous!

Make a dozen copies of the above contract and sign one each day.

Breakfast

MENU	PROTEIN	GRAIN	FRUIT or VEGETABLE
Pancakes and Sausage	(2 to 3 ozs.) One patty or two small links, try veggie!	1, 4-inch pancake or 4, 1-inch pancakes	Choice: blueberries (½ cup), bananas, strawberries, peaches. Crush ¼ cup in a blender and make fruit syrup!

- To drink, you may have coffee or tea, with a shot of milk in it, and a teaspoon of sugar if you wish.

- Don't forget—drink a big glass (eight to ten ounce) of water with your breakfast.

- Enjoy a moment of silence before you eat, appreciating all you have and realizing that feeding yourself is serious, important, and joyous. Then, eat slowly, savoring and enjoying each bite.

- Make sure to wait twenty minutes after your last bite to feel satisfied. You will feel that you've had enough.

Mid-Morning Snack

MENU	PROTEIN	GRAIN	FRUIT or VEGETABLE
Quesidilla (wrap)	Shredded cheese, melted (1½ ozs.)	Flour tortilla	Chopped tomato and green chillies (½ cup)

- DRINK: One large (eight to ten ounce) glass of water.

Lunch

MENU	PROTEIN	GRAIN	FRUIT or VEGETABLE
Sandwich: peanut butter and jelly	Peanut butter (⅓ cup)	One slice bread (or skip the grain part of your next snack and have two)	Fruit spread (¼ cup), unsweetened, preferably

- DRINK: One large (eight to ten ounce) glass of water.

Afternoon Snack

MENU	PROTEIN	GRAIN	FRUIT or VEGETABLE
		One slice bread (or skip it if you had it at lunch)	Fruit "roll-up" (sometimes called "leather")

- DRINK: One large (eight to ten ounce) glass of water.

Go bowling! Bowl with some friends after work, at least one twenty-minute game. If not, then speed-walk for five blocks one way and five blocks back.

PRAYER AND MEDITATION

Take five minutes for silent meditation. End with: "God, if it be your will, give me the will and strength to make little commitments to be the best person I can be for you every second of this day."

Day Twenty-Two

This is the beginning of the fourth week. Congratulations!

TODAY'S JOYOUS THOUGHT: *Let It Be!*

Remember the Beatles' beautiful song, "Let It Be"? Hum a few bars and sing a few words if you can. "When I find myself in times of trouble, Mother Mary comes to me, speaking words of wisdom, let it be...."

Those really are true words of wisdom: spiritual wisdom. Let it be. If you find yourself in trouble, go to God (as you know Him or Her), then let it be.

Let it be—let the problem surface, analyze it, and plan a course of action—then get over it. In other words: move on. Don't let the problem fester or it will grow larger and unmanageable. I believe God gives us problems as gifts. They're tough love surprises, but never too much to handle. I also believe that challenges and troubles are ways that motivate us to remember to go to God for help.

DO THIS TODAY

Here's a twist that'll help you a lot. Challenge yourself to actually *not* work on a problem today! Just let it be! Stop worrying about it. Don't drop everything and attack it. Just live with it for a day. Give it a rest. Don't try to solve it yourself for a change.

Take the extra time to ask for spiritual help. Hand the problem to God through prayer and ask for Him to reveal what to do with it... if anything. The answer may be to just let it be.

As this day is a new beginning (like every day, of course), it's also the beginning of a new food week. It's a special day. This is the day you begin to be completely on The Joy of Weight Loss Eating Plan. Hopefully, you've acclimated yourself fairly well to the previous meals and snacks and perhaps eaten less for dinner and the evening snack already. Either way, OK, here we go! Let's celebrate and really enjoy eating!

Breakfast

M E N U	PROTEIN	GRAIN	FRUIT or VEGETABLE
French toast	2 eggs for the batter dip	Bread (1 slice)	Add a topping of fruit, chopped (½ cup)

- To drink, you may have coffee or tea, with a shot of milk in it, and a teaspoon of sugar if you wish.

- Don't forget—drink a big glass (eight to ten ounce) of water with your breakfast.

- Enjoy a moment of silence before you eat, appreciating all you have and realizing that feeding yourself is serious, important, and joyous. Then, eat slowly, savoring and enjoying each bite.

- Make sure to wait twenty minutes after your last bite to feel satisfied. You will feel that you've had enough.

Mid-Morning Snack

Protein with this snack; none this afternoon. You should have your vegetable now, because you had fruit this morning. Fruit again for lunch.

M E N U	PROTEIN	GRAIN	FRUIT or VEGETABLE
Turkey roll-up	Turkey breast (2 to 3 ozs.)	Bread (1 slice)	Vegetable juice (¾ cup)

- DRINK: One large (eight to ten ounce) glass of water.

Lunch

M E N U	PROTEIN	GRAIN	FRUIT or VEGETABLE
Salad: fruit and cottage cheese	Cottage cheese (1½ ozs.)	Whole wheat bread (1 slice)	Fresh peach, orange, apple, pear, banana slices (1 medium or ½ cup), chopped

- DRINK: One large (eight to ten ounce) glass of water.

Afternoon Snack

No protein now, since you had it for the morning snack.

MENU	PROTEIN	GRAIN	FRUIT or VEGETABLE
Cornbread and tomato juice	None	Cornbread one 2-inch slice	(¾ cup) tomato juice— add some hot sauce, or Worcester sauce if you dare!

- **DRINK: One large (eight to ten ounce) glass of water.**

Dinner

It's a simple concept, dinner. Same three-group combination, one serving from each:

- **A protein (meat or dairy group, alternating)**

- **A grain**

- **A vegetable or fruit (alternating)**

- **One large (eight to ten ounce) glass of water.**

PROTEIN

You have had two servings from the meat protein group so far today (eggs for breakfast, turkey for the mid-morning snack), and one serving from the dairy protein group (cottage cheese at lunch). Therefore, because you need two servings from each group, you are due another dairy group serving at dinner tonight.

VEGETABLE AND FRUIT

You have had wonderfully alternating fruits and vegetables for breakfast (fruit), mid-morning snack (vegetable), lunch (fruit) and afternoon snack (vegetable)—what more is left? If you guessed vegetable, you get ten joyous points! That's because you're supposed to have three servings per day of vegetables.

MENU	PROTEIN	GRAIN	FRUIT or VEGETABLE
Lasagna	Ground beef or veggie protein and shredded cheese (2 ozs.)	Pasta: cooked lasagna noodles (½ cup)	Tomato sauce (¾ cup)

- **DRINK: One large (eight to ten ounce) glass of water.**

Evening Snack (two hours after dinner, two hours before bed)

If you've eaten enough during the day, have a light snack of only a grain after dinner. If you are missing some servings of a fruit or vegetable, the after-dinner snack is a great time to make up and get them covered. Skip the meat or dairy protein unless you absolutely must. If you've eaten too much, you may occasionally cut out the evening snack all together, but I don't recommend it often. I encourage you to have a little something two hours before bedtime, just to keep your body nourished through the night. But don't do it right before bed, however, or you may get digestion problems!

Today, we got everything from all the food groups in fairly well. What's missing is only a grain. If you really want, you could have another serving of vegetables or fruit (juice, perhaps) and it won't hurt. That's because vegetables and fruits are low in fats. I would not recommend having another serving of protein, however. It's too heavy and too much fat right before bed.

MENU	PROTEIN	GRAIN	FRUIT or VEGETABLE
	None	Whole wheat crackers	Juice, if you crave it—fruit or vegetable (¾ cup)

- **DRINK: One large (eight to ten ounce) glass of water.**

TODAY'S ACTIVITY

This being the fourth week, you're ready to ascend to another pinnacle of movement and activity—adding merely ten more minutes to your activity plan today, bringing you up to thirty minutes will do it.

You can do the thirty minutes all at once, or split it up into ten-minute intervals. The point is to to move every day. You could do a half-hour joyful walk in the park at dawn.

Or you could:

- **Walk for ten minutes in the morning with the dog. (Don't just watch, walk!)**
- **Then work out for twenty minutes during lunch: jumping, stretching, twisting, dancing to music.**

Or make up your own thirty-minute routine. Just make certain that it's enjoyable, and that you do it for sure.

Congratulations. This is what The Joy of Weight Loss Eating and Activity plans are all about! Eat and move like this for the rest of your life and you will always be healthy and never worry about your weight again. Thank God!

And speaking of God . . .

PRAYER AND MEDITATION: *Rising Above, Letting It Be*

Today, to celebrate your fourth week, here's a very special, very powerful meditation.

Go to your private sacred space, get quiet and peaceful, and still your mind of any and all thoughts.... Breathe out and in, slowly, deeply, ten times....

Picture a problem or concern you have in your mind. Really see it clearly. If it's another person, see them in your mind's eye. If it's money, picture currency, bills, or account statements; if it's tangible property, picture it. If it's just a worry about the future, try your best to see it and make it mentally real.

Now picture yourself magically, joyously floating above the pictured problem. You're flying in mid-air, higher and higher. Let out a laugh as you let your cares drift away, below you. Wave goodbye to them! Rise above and beyond the problem(s). Higher and higher! Further and further rising above, until you no longer see them.

Now take a few minutes to let yourself be in this transcendent, floating mental heaven. Take in a few sighs of relief and joy. Don't worry, everything's going to be all right. Now come back to earth. A few more deep breaths. Slowly open your eyes. You've let your problems be, and risen above them—at least for a few minutes.

Day Twenty-Three ⌒

TODAY'S JOYOUS THOUGHT: *Sincerity*

The next truth about losing weight, connected to letting it be, is the importance of being completely sincere. If you let yourself be totally real, honest, and sincere in all of your endeavors and with others, your life will be much easier. You may or may not at first think that this has anything to do with losing weight, but once you realize the power of sincerity, you will see that it has everything to do with it.

You may have been living under an illusion. You may well have been unknowingly telling yourself lies to avoid having to deal with the difficulty of your life.

As we discussed in earlier parts of this book, you may have been protecting yourself by making yourself fat. You could have been overfeeding over and over again because it seemed easier at the time. The pain of facing the side-effects of overeating and inactivity was too great to bear. The truths of your life, your greatest fears and self-hatred, were what you had—so you hung onto them. You may have been instinctively avoiding the pain of living. You could have been under a really grand illusion or fantasy that everything in life is supposed to be pleasurable and easy. This just isn't so. This may be a little difficult to hear, but sometimes the truth hurts.

The truth can also set you free, truly. Perhaps the greatest illusion of all is that the pain and sorrow of life is unbearable. The sincere truth is that life is actually quite livable once you sincerely face it little by little, step by step. You do your best, be your real self, and let God guide you. In doing these things, your illusions and self-destruction slowly and surely fade away over time as you and God heal them by allowing yourself to be completely and sincerely yourself.

DO THIS TODAY

Commit to God and yourself to be honest and real today. Express your true feelings, as long as they won't hurt someone else. Tell someone what's really going on in you. Put away the mask and let your true self show through.

TODAY'S MENU

Breakfast

MENU	PROTEIN	GRAIN	FRUIT or VEGETABLE
A bowl of cereal	Milk (1 cup)	Cereal (1 oz., about ½ cup average)	Banana, cut-up

- To drink, you may have coffee or tea, with a shot of milk in it, and a teaspoon of sugar if you wish.

- Don't forget—drink a big glass (eight to ten ounce) of water with your breakfast.

- Enjoy a moment of silence before you eat, appreciating all you have and realizing that feeding yourself is serious, important, and joyous. Then, eat slowly, savoring and enjoying each bite.

- Make sure to wait twenty minutes after your last bite to feel satisfied. You will feel that you've had enough.

Mid-Morning Snack

Notice we're having two fruits and two dairy proteins in a row. You may do that! This is a cold salad dish, that you might pick up from a supermarket salad bar, or a left-over. Ultimately, we want you to have what you feel like having—your own informed choice—and not just follow your diet from a book!

M E N U	PROTEIN	GRAIN	FRUIT or VEGETABLE
Pasta Florentine	Diced mozzarella (2 ozs.)	Pasta shells, cooked (½ cup)	Cooked spinach and garlic (in the pasta)

- **DRINK: One large (eight to ten ounce) glass of water.**

Lunch

Time to have a different protein group, for the sake of variety and balance.

M E N U	PROTEIN	GRAIN	FRUIT or VEGETABLE
Turkey chili	Turkey cubes, or TVP* (textured veg. protein) kidney beans (2 to 3 ozs.)	Cornbread (2 x 2-inch square)	Cooked corn, tomatillos, tomatoes, black olives (½ cup)

- **DRINK: One large (eight to ten ounce) glass of water.**

Afternoon Snack

Remember, only one protein at snack time, per day. We'll skip it now.

M E N U	PROTEIN	GRAIN	FRUIT or VEGETABLE
	None	Melba toast (2 small slices)	Tangerine (medium)

- **DRINK: One large (eight to ten ounce) glass of water.**

Dinner

We only had one meat group (at lunch), but have had two dairy group servings (breakfast and mid-morning snack). So, time for another meat group. Also, we're due another vegetable. Fruits are taken care of for the day, today.

M E N U	PROTEIN	GRAIN	FRUIT or VEGETABLE
Thai shrimp and vegetables	Cooked shrimp and chopped peanut, in sauce (2 ozs.)	Thai "glass" noodles (½ cup)	Scallions, snow peas, shredded carrot (½ cup)

- **DRINK: One large (eight to ten ounce) glass of water.**

Evening Snack

Had enough proteins, fruits, and vegetables. Need only one more grain group serving to make it six. Another perfect, delicious day! It's really not hard to eat healthy, is it?

MENU	PROTEIN	GRAIN	FRUIT or VEGETABLE
	None	Parkerhouse dinner roll (1)	None

- **DRINK: One large (eight to ten ounce) glass of water.**

TODAY'S ACTIVITY

The minutes are thirty, don't be afraid to get dirty! Climb a tree. Hike in the woods; go barefooted! Wade in a stream. Roll in the grass. Get out and get happy!

PRAYER AND MEDITATION

Take five minutes for silent meditation, before you begin your day today. Then, revel in reality just before bed tonight. Appreciate yourself for taking the leap of faith and not giving up. Thank yourself for speaking your truth and having the courage to begin to be totally real today.

Just before you fall asleep, say this prayer: "God, if it be thy will, grant me the personal integrity to be completely myself. With your grace, let me put aside my illusions, fears, self-hatred, and destructive ways. I didn't mean to hurt myself! I just didn't know any better. I love you God. Thank you for everything. Amen."

TODAY'S JOYOUS THOUGHT: *Friendship*

We humans are creatures of community. We just do not do well alone. It seems like we are born to work together, in cooperation. Some of us are good at certain things but not others. It takes all of us together, in community, in friendship, to build, operate, and create.

. . . in a study reported in the American Journal of Epidemiology *of nearly seven thousand men and Women between the age of thirty and sixty-nine in Alameda County, California, researchers found that social isolation has pervasive health consequences.*

When I weighed a lot, I was alone a lot. I had a couple of friends, some really *true* friends, but most of the time I was alone in front of the TV or locked in my room listening to music. Since I felt ashamed to be seen in public, I preferred to be alone. I felt bad, so I ate to feel better, which made me even fatter. I hope you're not that way. I pray that no one has to be alone and ashamed, anymore. I know, however, that many overweight people are alone and lonely. It doesn't have to be that way. We don't have to be without friends.

DO THIS TODAY

Connect with a friend—either an old, true friend, or make a new one. You could call a friend you haven't spoken with in a long time. Just catch up, talk small talk, share concerns, open up and tell a secret if you feel trusting enough. Get together to walk, eat a healthy meal, see a movie, go bowling, play ball, or go shopping. Talk about the joys in your life. Talk about the challenges and hardships and what action you're taking to cope or improve them. Tell them about this program and the increasing joy you're experiencing—in losing weight!

Or make a new friend. Here's how: strike up a conversation about them. Ask them about a book they're reading, or a painting on the wall, a picture on their shelf, or the sure-fire conversation-starter question: "Where are you from?" Be genuinely interested. Ask questions. Find a common interest between you in a situation you're both in, or where there's work to be done, or you have concerns about something (politics, the economy, fashion, spirituality, architecture, current fiction or non-fiction, movies, music, technology...). It's an endlessly interesting world! Everyone wants to have a friend— they're simply waiting for someone to show the slightest interest in them. Just like you are!

How nice it would be to share a meal with a friend, today.

Breakfast

M E N U	PROTEIN	GRAIN	FRUIT or VEGETABLE
Waffles and ham	Ham—meat or veggie (2 oz. slice)	Waffle	Fruit syrup/spread, unsweetened (½ cup)

- To drink, you may have coffee or tea, with a shot of milk in it, and a teaspoon of sugar if you wish.
- Don't forget—drink a big glass (eight to ten ounce) of water with your breakfast.
- Enjoy a moment of silence before you eat, appreciating all you have and realizing that feeding yourself is serious, important, and joyous. Then, eat slowly, savoring and enjoying each bite.
- Make sure to wait twenty minutes after your last bite to feel satisfied. You will feel that you've had enough.

Mid-Morning Snack

Yesterday, you had protein in the morning. For the sake of variety, have the once daily snack protein this afternoon, unless you're craving it now. If so, have it!

M E N U	PROTEIN	GRAIN	FRUIT or VEGETABLE
Five Greek dolma (stuffed grape leaves) and olives	None	Rice, in the grape leaves (about ½ cup)	Grape leaves (approx. ½ cup), green olives (¼ cup)

- DRINK: One large (eight to ten ounce) glass of water.

Lunch

M E N U	PROTEIN	GRAIN	FRUIT or VEGETABLE
Hamburger or veggie burger	Patty—beef, turkey or veggie (2 ozs.)	Small bun	Lettuce and tomato, pickles on the side, ketchup or mustard if you like.

- DRINK: One large (eight to ten ounce) glass of water.

Afternoon Snack

Have the snack protein now, because you didn't this morning. You've had a fruit for breakfast, then two vegetables for snack and lunch. This is an example of saving up the second of two fruit servings for either dinner or evening snack.

MENU	PROTEIN	GRAIN	FRUIT or VEGETABLE
	Brie cheese, natural (1½ oz.)	Oat-bran or graham crackers (5, average)	None

- **DRINK: One large (eight to ten ounce) glass of water.**

Dinner

You had two meat proteins already today (satisfying that requirement), and one dairy. You're due another dairy to make it two in that protein group. You've had one fruit and two vegetables, so you're due another fruit (two a day) and a vegetable (three a day) for dinner or evening snack. Getting the hang of it?

MENU	PROTEIN	GRAIN	FRUIT or VEGETABLE
Grilled cheese sandwich	Cheddar or American cheese (2 slices)	Whole wheat or rye bread (1 slice), or skip the grain part of your next snack and have two	Strawberries (½ cup)

- **DRINK: One large (eight to ten ounce) glass of water.**

Evening Snack

If you had two slices of bread, that completed your grains for the day. If you had the strawberries, that completed your fruit servings for the day. You have a choice:

- **If you're not hungry, don't eat!**
- **If you are, you may go ahead...**
- **A grain (bread, crackers, rice, leftover pasta or rice)**
- **Or fruit or vegetable (apple, orange, banana, cucumber, sweet potato, plantain)**

Be conscious, however, that you would be eating more than necessary for weight loss. This is a time when you may need a little more food, and that's OK as long as you're in control and making conscious decisions. If it's a binge, ask God for help. If you're regularly overeating or bingeing, then seek help from a doctor.

- **DRINK: One large (eight to ten ounce) glass of water.**

TODAY'S ACTIVITY

Why not exercise for thirty minutes today with a friend? Make a regular weekly or twice weekly (or more!) time to have fun together. I have been playing racquetball and squash with my friend Jamahl once a week for over six years! We aren't very good at it, but we sure have fun and work up a lot of sweat without even thinking! I wouldn't miss that time together for anything. My wife Catherine and I like to go to aerobics, rebounding, and body-works classes often, too. We goof around and joke during the wildly joyous sessions.

PRAYER AND MEDITATION

Take five minutes for silent meditation.

"God, I'm so fortunate to have my friends. My friends save me, and I love them. May I be as good a friend to them as they are to me. Amen."

Day Twenty-Five

TODAY'S JOYOUS THOUGHT: *The Joy of Working*

Give your work all you've got. Throw yourself into it, even doing a little extra if you can. Your work is your livelihood, your purpose, and your mission in life.

If you possibly can, love your work. Make it joyous by getting into it. The best kind of work is the kind that not only helps you but helps others as well. You make a living and your work enriches your fellow humans.

If you are not working, by all means do anything you can to get involved and participate in life. If you don't need the money, then volunteer at something. If you can't find a job or no one will hire you, get help from a job counselor. There's a job for everyone. You just have to be open to it.

People who aren't working or are in a job that's unfulfilling or demeaning need to change their situation immediately. If that's you, it could be a major cause of your weight problem. It's vitally important to work and to find joy in working.

Write down your mission statement. Think about what's important to you in terms of career or profession, job, money, service to others, spiritual contribution, social functioning, learning, emotional and intellectual satisfaction, and what your goal as a human being is. Lastly, in your personal mission statement, explore how you get joy from your work and what you could do to build and amplify that joy.

TODAY'S MENU

Breakfast

MENU	PROTEIN	GRAIN	FRUIT or VEGETABLE
Fruit yogurt and toast	Yogurt (1 cup)	Slice of toast	Chopped pineapple (½ cup)

- To drink, you may have coffee or tea, with a shot of milk in it, and a teaspoon of sugar if you wish.

- Don't forget—drink a big glass (eight to ten ounce) of water with your breakfast.

- Enjoy a moment of silence before you eat, appreciating all you have and realizing that feeding yourself is serious, important, and joyous. Then, eat slowly, savoring and enjoying each bite.

- Make sure to wait twenty minutes after your last bite to feel satisfied. You will feel that you've had enough

Mid-Morning Snack

MENU	PROTEIN	GRAIN	FRUIT or VEGETABLE
	Turkey (2 to 3 ozs.)	Baked corn chips (10)	Apple (medium)

- DRINK: One large (eight to ten ounce) glass of water.

Lunch

Take a break from meat and dairy and have vegetable protein in the form of beans for lunch. It's a really tasty and healthy way to go.

M E N U	PROTEIN	GRAIN	FRUIT or VEGETABLE
Salad bar	Beans: chick, kidney, canoli, black-eyed (½ cup)	Croutons (½ cup)	Leafy greens (¾ cup), add chopped, mixed vegetables: carrot, beets, radishes, cucumber, tomato, zucchini, etc. (¼ cup)

- **DRINK: One large (eight to ten ounce) glass of water.**

Afternoon Snack

M E N U	PROTEIN	GRAIN	FRUIT or VEGETABLE
Vegetable soup	None	Onion or sesame bagel (½)	Mixed vegetables in a vegetable broth (½ cup)

- **DRINK: One large (eight to ten ounce) glass of water.**

Dinner

M E N U	PROTEIN	GRAIN	FRUIT or VEGETABLE
Pasta primavera	Grated Parmesan cheese (2 ozs.)	Pasta, try angel hair (½ cup, cooked)	Chopped vegetables: carrots, broccoli, spinach, onions, green beans, squash (½ cup)

- **DRINK: One large (eight to ten ounce) glass of water.**

Evening Snack:

M E N U	PROTEIN	GRAIN	FRUIT or VEGETABLE
	None	Matzo—unleavened bread (1 slice)	Grapes (½ cup)

- **DRINK: One large (eight to ten ounce) glass of water.**

TODAY'S ACTIVITY

Thirty minutes, at work! Sign up for a corporate workout. Take a beginners group. Many companies have free or low-cost programs or personal trainers at your disposal. If your company does not, ask your boss to set one up. After all, at work workouts help everyone involved: employees get happier and healthier, have fewer sick days, more energy, and better moods. That's great for employers, too.

While at work, take time to rest and recharge, spiritually. Take a one-minute meditation or emergency-calmer by going into a spare room (or a restroom stall) and close your eyes. Be silent and still. Breathe deep. Say a prayer of gratitude to God for the ability to work and for your livelihood and purpose in life.

Day Twenty-Six

TODAY'S JOYOUS THOUGHT: *Understanding*

The more you know about yourself and the world, the better. It pays to sharpen your intellect and collect knowledge. Remember the advertising phrase, "a mind is a terrible thing to waste." Life gets easier the more you know about it.

Someone also once said: "A waist is a terrible thing to mind!" It will help your weight loss program if you continue to understand why you're overweight, what's available to help you, and what others have done. Every time a new research study comes out, get it and read it. There have been many major contributions to understanding in the last ten years, such as discovery of a gene that causes a predisposition to obesity (the OB gene). Studies like this help you understand that your obesity is not necessarily due to your bad habits entirely—you may have an unfortunate genetic, family predisposition. Reading the statistics on obesity can really motivate you to keep up the good work. Knowing that just even being slightly overweight significantly increases your risk of fatal illness—such as coronary heart disease, cancer, arthritis, and many others—may also keep convincing you to hold off on those extra bites.

Reading spiritual and philosophical books and inspirational stories is also greatly enriching. A good idea can really brighten your day and light your way through your life journey.

DO THIS TODAY

Look for greater knowledge and understanding at a library or search the Internet for information. Take time to read an article in a periodical or a passage from a book.

It would also be a good idea today to again return to your food logs from the first week. Study the connections between emotions and eating, and take another look at the amount of food you used to eat compared to how much you're eating now. You may be very surprised. Also, try to look at other factors such as what time you ate, where, what you were doing at the time or just before that may have prompted you to overeat. Also look at the types of food: Were you getting all of the five food groups in? This information may be very illuminating. It may be of further use to read more about weight management, the psychology of obesity, nutrition, behavior research, or recreation.

TODAY'S MENU

Breakfast

M E N U	PROTEIN	GRAIN	FRUIT or VEGETABLE
Sausage biscuit	Sausage, meat or veggie (2 to 3 oz.)	Biscuit	Orange juice (¾ cup)

- To drink, you may have coffee or tea, with a shot of milk in it, and a teaspoon of sugar if you wish.

- Don't forget—drink a big glass (eight to ten ounce) of water with your breakfast.

- Enjoy a moment of silence before you eat, appreciating all you have and realizing that feeding yourself is serious, important, and joyous. Then, eat slowly, savoring and enjoying each bite.

- Make sure to wait twenty minutes after your last bite to feel satisfied. You will feel that you've had enough.

Mid-Morning Snack

M E N U	PROTEIN	GRAIN	FRUIT or VEGETABLE
Muffin and fruit		Small muffin	Fruit cup (½ cup)

- DRINK: One large (eight to ten ounce) glass of water.

Lunch

M E N U	PROTEIN	GRAIN	FRUIT or VEGETABLE
Spanish roast chicken	Roasted chicken, spicy herb marinade (2 to 3 ozs.)	Yellow rice (½ cup)	Mixed vegetables, cooked —plantain, green olive, tomato, hot peppers. (½ cup)

- DRINK: One large (eight to ten ounce) glass of water.

Afternoon Snack

MENU	PROTEIN	GRAIN	FRUIT or VEGETABLE
Crudités with dip	Pea or bean dip —chick peas, black or kidney beans mashed (½ cup, in ½ cup yogurt)		Mixed into dip: shredded carrots, cucumbers, radishes, Tabasco or jalapeno sauce (½ cup total)

- **DRINK: One large (eight to ten ounce) glass of water.**

Dinner

MENU	PROTEIN	GRAIN	FRUIT or VEGETABLE
Russian dinner	Cheese blintzes	Kasha (boiled seasoned bulgur wheat grain or substitute cooked barley or tabouli salad)	Borscht (beet soup, cold or hot) with small potato

- **DRINK: One large (eight to ten ounce) glass of water.**

Evening Snack

You've satisfied your meat proteins (two) for the day, but you've only had one of two for dairy protein. You've satisfied all of your vegetables (three) and fruits (two). All that's left is a grain. Enjoy!

MENU	PROTEIN	GRAIN	FRUIT or VEGETABLE
	None	Belgian wafers (5 small, average)	None

- **DRINK: One large (eight to ten ounce) glass of water.**

TODAY'S ACTIVITY

Park your car four or five blocks away from your destination and then walk for thirty minutes to where you're going. Do this no matter what the weather is. Weather is enjoyable if you're prepared for it with the proper clothing, rain gear, boots, or coat. It sure keeps you from being bored!

Take five minutes for silent meditation. Then ask for help again today, through prayer and spiritual communion.

"God, teach me to teach myself. Let me learn everything I can about your wondrous creation. If it be Your will, let me learn about myself and my amazing life. Let me never stop learning. Grant me continued interest in new facts and truths and not fear what they may mean to me. Amen."

Day Twenty-Seven

TODAY'S JOYOUS THOUGHT: *Helping Others Helps Me*

When you give a little of yourself to help someone else, it's a double bonus. You actually help yourself in the process. By stepping outside yourself and extending, you cause yourself to grow beyond your own shell. Your compassion and empathy grows. Understanding of human emotions and problems deepens as you hear them from another point of view. You realize you're not alone, and that others may have a harder life than you do. You get a sense of joy in assisting someone's accomplishment of their challenges and a new perspective on your own. You're able to see your own problems reflected in someone else's life, without your emotional hindrances getting in the way. You temporarily put your troubles aside to care for another person.

You feel powerful and useful, valuable and great, because you're looked up to. Rewards and personal satisfaction are bountiful for both of you, as you see God in the other.

DO THIS TODAY

Do something wonderful for someone, today—something unexpected, a nice word, an offer to help, or a smile of understanding.

TODAY'S MENU

Breakfast

MENU	PROTEIN	GRAIN	FRUIT or VEGETABLE
A bowl of cereal	Milk (1 cup)	Cereal (1 oz., about ¾ cup average)	Banana, cut-up

- To drink, you may have coffee or tea, with a shot of milk in it, and a teaspoon of sugar if you wish.

- Don't forget—drink a big glass (eight to ten ounce) of water with your breakfast.

- Enjoy a moment of silence before you eat, appreciating all you have and realizing that feeding yourself is serious, important, and joyous. Then, eat slowly, savoring and enjoying each bite.

- Make sure to wait twenty minutes after your last bite to feel satisfied. You will feel that you've had enough.

Mid-Morning Snack

M E N U	PROTEIN	GRAIN	FRUIT or VEGETABLE
	None	Pretzels (7 small, 2 big)	Cherry tomatoes (½ cup)

- DRINK: One large (eight to ten ounce) glass of water.

Lunch

You don't always have to have a different meal. Leftovers are just fine! Notice it's *fried* chicken. Yes, I think it's OK to have fried food once in a while, like once a week, while losing weight.

M E N U	PROTEIN	GRAIN	FRUIT or VEGETABLE
Leftover chicken	Fried chicken, thigh or breast (about 2 ozs.)	Biscuit	Coleslaw

- DRINK: One large (eight to ten ounce) glass of water.

Afternoon Snack

M E N U	PROTEIN	GRAIN	FRUIT or VEGETABLE
		Mini pretzel sticks	Honey tangerine

- DRINK: One large (eight to ten ounce) glass of water.

Dinner

Notice two vegetables, here. Why not? (This will then satisfy the three for the day.)

M E N U	PROTEIN	GRAIN	FRUIT or VEGETABLE
Salmon	Broiled salmon with dill and lemon (2 ozs.)	French bread (1 slice)	Baked potato (medium) Broccoli (about ½ cup)

- **DRINK: One large (eight to ten ounce) glass of water.**

Evening Snack

M E N U	PROTEIN	GRAIN	FRUIT or VEGETABLE
	Yogurt (I cup)	Granola mixed in (¼ cup)	

- **DRINK: One large (eight to ten ounce) glass of water.**

TODAY'S ACTIVITY

Stretch for five minutes in your living room. Put on a CD or music videos and dance to music for twenty minutes. Go wild! Then stretch and cool down for another five minutes.

PRAYER AND MEDITATION

This is a practical meditation. Find someone and offer to listen to their problems for ten minutes today. Sit down together and listen without any comments, analysis, or interruptions. When they're done, say: "I understand what you mean, and I can see how you feel that way."

Be sure to take five minutes for your silent meditation.

Day Twenty-Eight

TODAY'S JOYOUS THOUGHT: *Surrendering the Self-Destruction*

Every time I ran for comfort foods, like downing a dozen donuts or shoving a box of chocolate sandwich cookies in my mouth as fast as I could, I would always wonder why I couldn't stop. The compulsion had me. I had to have some pleasurable relief and had to have it *now*. For years, my self-destructive behaviors were a mystery. Sure, I knew I was hurting myself, but that didn't matter in times of crisis. Why I didn't care was beyond me. If my car broke down, I would first think of the nearest restaurant or snack bar, not a mechanic shop. If I had a bad day at school or work, I would use cupcakes or candy to soothe the pain instead of taking action to fix the problem. When I was lonely, I'd go for brownies instead of companionship.

Once I gave my unsolvable eating mystery to God and began to receive His help, things slowly became clear. I felt afraid. I felt alone and unloved. But I wasn't conscious of that pain and self-hate, only of the destructive behavior that I couldn't control.

You can also unlock the mysteries behind your vices by quieting down your mind in times of crisis and letting God help you get honest with yourself. Self-destructive behavior is often a need to love and be loved due to old self-hatred. Feel God's unconditional love for you, begin to accept His love through others, and the self-hatred and self-abusive vices will eventually melt away.

DO THIS TODAY

Take ten minutes, now or before the day is done, to get quiet and write down five moments of self-destructive behavior you've recently experienced. Then probe a little deeper and think about what you were going through and feeling just before you overate or didn't take care of yourself. If you don't instantly understand your triggering emotions, that's OK for now. It takes time. Ask God for help with this. Then the next time you're about to self-destruct with food—stop, say a prayer ("God, Help me, please!"), and see if there's something upsetting you. It could be a big, obvious thing, or something really little and seemingly irrelevant. By just taking an extra moment to get behind the behavior, you're already half the way to finding liberation from its grip on you.

TODAY'S MENU

Breakfast

M E N U	PROTEIN	GRAIN	FRUIT or VEGETABLE
Grilled Cheese bagel	Cheese, natural (1½ oz.), processed (2 ozs., about two slices)	Small bagel, toasted (with cheese melted)	Grilled vegetables: onions, tomato, peppers, mushrooms (½ cup)

- To drink, you may have coffee or tea, with a shot of milk in it, and a teaspoon of sugar if you wish.

- Don't forget—drink a big glass (eight to ten ounce) of water with your breakfast.

- Enjoy a moment of silence before you eat, appreciating all you have and realizing that feeding yourself is serious, important, and joyous. Then, eat slowly, savoring and enjoying each bite.

- Make sure to wait twenty minutes after your last bite to feel satisfied. You will feel that you've had enough.

Mid-Morning Snack

M E N U	PROTEIN	GRAIN	FRUIT or VEGETABLE
	Peanuts (2 tbs)	Popcorn (1 cup, approx., not buttered)	Apple juice (¾ cup)

- DRINK: One large (eight to ten ounce) glass of water.

Lunch

M E N U	PROTEIN	GRAIN	FRUIT or VEGETABLE
Wrap: Turkey breast	Turkey breast (2 or 3 ozs. sliced)	Flour tortilla (1)	Shredded lettuce, sliced tomato and dill pickles (½ cup)

- DRINK: One large (eight to ten ounce) glass of water.

Afternoon Snack

M E N U	PROTEIN	GRAIN	FRUIT or VEGETABLE
		Cornbread (2 x 2-inch square)	

- DRINK: One large (eight to ten ounce) glass of water.

Dinner

M E N U	PROTEIN	GRAIN	FRUIT or VEGETABLE
Italian eggplant Parmesan	Mozzarella cheese, melted on top (1½ ozs.)	Garlic bread (1 slice), with butter and one clove crushed garlic (½ teaspoon)	Eggplant slices (½ cup), lightly sautéed in one tsp. olive oil, tomato sauce.

- DRINK: One large (eight to ten ounce) glass of water.

Evening Snack

M E N U	PROTEIN	GRAIN	FRUIT or VEGETABLE
		2 bread sticks	Hot vegetable soup (½ cup)

- DRINK: One large (eight to ten ounce) glass of water.

Thirty minutes at a playground, with a kid! Climb the jungle gym, swing on swings, push the merry-go-round, hang on the parallel bars, pull yourself up on the rings, skip rope, play hop-scotch.

PRAYER AND MEDITATION

Get down on your knees and bow your head to the ground again. Thank God for your life, then tell Him that you will rely on Him 100 percent, no matter what may come. Ask Him for guidance, particularly when you're about to overeat or can't get up out of the chair. Tell God that you believe in Him and love Him.

Then, as we do every day, take some time to be totally still and quiet, for at least five minutes; more if possible.

Day Twenty-Nine

TODAY'S JOYOUS THOUGHT: *Maintaining Day by Day*

Relax in the knowledge that you're doing your best, that quality takes time, and keep giving yourself gifts of change. This is a whole new solution; it isn't just a weight loss diet such as you've been on before. While you may want or expect to drop five or more pounds in one week and you probably did in the past on fad diets, this program is different. God can help you actually keep the weight off, if you want it enough. God will enable you to stick with it long enough to let new habits become instinctual.

The goal is to find and maintain a healthy, reasonable weight, and not just lose it. You do that by finding true happiness and joy with God and becoming a whole person experiencing life in every way. You do it by following your food plan and eating one serving at a time. And you move and actively use your body every day. Consistently give yourself these three gifts—and the weight will come off slowly but steadily.

As I've said, when shedding pounds, a good, safe average rate over time is between one to two pounds per week, or four to eight pounds a month. But you won't know it immediately after just one week. *Don't get on a scale until the end of the first month.* Promise yourself this. As a matter of fact, don't judge your progress by weight alone. Don't depend on people saying "You look really thin." Adopt some new standards of success: see if you feel better. Check if you have a little more energy, feel lighter, get into your clothes a little easier. Trust in God that you are working with Him to solve the problem. Do your part every day, then leave the results to Him.

Relax: you're going to be OK. Keep working. Your efforts are working. Take your time, and make another commitment to keep up the good work. Today is a good day to strengthen your commitment by reminding yourself of your priorities. Take five minutes right now to answer the following questions. Really search your heart and be completely honest.

"I want to manage my weight because I am concerned about

_____."

"Although I may not feel important sometimes, I am trying to show myself that I care by

_____."

(List two or more specific things you're doing or want to do to feel better).

"In the past, I have worked hard, had patience, and was rewarded with

_____."

TODAY'S MENU

Breakfast

MENU	PROTEIN	GRAIN	FRUIT or VEGETABLE
Pancakes and sausage	Try veggie (2 to 3 ozs. (1 patty, or 2 small links)	1, 4-inch pancake or 4, 1-inch pancakes	Choice: blueberries, bananas, strawberries, peaches.

- To drink, you may have coffee or tea, with a shot of milk in it, and a teaspoon of sugar if you wish.

- Don't forget—drink a big glass (eight to ten ounce) of water with your breakfast.

- Enjoy a moment of silence before you eat, appreciating all you have and realizing that feeding yourself is serious, important, and joyous. Then, eat slowly, savoring and enjoying each bite.

- Make sure to wait twenty minutes after your last bite to feel satisfied. You will feel that you've had enough.

Mid-Morning Snack

This is what you could do if you're ravenously hungry this morning. Have a substantial snack and then plan to have less for lunch or dinner. Feel free to design variety into your food plan, by making it your own.

M E N U	PROTEIN	GRAIN	FRUIT or VEGETABLE
Strawberry yogurt banana split	Yogurt (½ cup) almonds, chopped, toasted (1 tbs)	Vanilla wafers (4, approx.)	Banana (½) Strawberries (¼ cup)

- **DRINK: One large (eight to ten ounce) glass of water.**

Lunch

This is a lighter lunch, if you're no longer as hungry since you had a bigger snack.

M E N U	PROTEIN	GRAIN	FRUIT or VEGETABLE
	Bouillon (1 cup)	Rolls (2) (note: this is two servings)	Applesauce (½ cup)

- **DRINK: One large (eight to ten ounce) glass of water.**

Afternoon Snack

M E N U	PROTEIN	GRAIN	FRUIT or VEGETABLE
	Chicken leg (1 average)	Biscuit	Coleslaw with vinegar dressing (½ cup)

- **DRINK: One large (eight to ten ounce) glass of water.**

Dinner:

Some folks like sushi, some don't. Have it if you do, and, if not, have cooked fish.

M E N U	PROTEIN	GRAIN	FRUIT or VEGETABLE
Japanese sushi	Fish: raw tuna, salmon, crab roll, mackerel (2 to 3 ozs.)	Japanese rice (½ cup in the rolled sushi)	Cucumber (½ cup) rolled in the sushi

- **DRINK: One large (eight to ten ounce) glass of water.**

Evening Snack

You have had all of your allotments for today of everything. Hopefully, you're not hungry. Skip the snack if possible. Drink a glass of water, or have some hot herbal tea before you turn over your burdens to God tonight.

PRAYER AND MEDITATION

"God, please give me the strength to be patient so that I can do your will at the right time. I'm learning that I may be expecting immediate big changes, and that's unrealistic. Now I just want to receive your help and take change as it comes, on your schedule. Most of all, if it be your will, please give me the desire and determination to make what I've learned a part of my life."

As a motivating challenge, see if you can stand in one place and do absolutely nothing for five minutes. Stand completely still—no movement, no looking, no thoughts, only breathing. Tell yourself that you're waiting and learning patience, then release all thoughts. Sound easy? Just try it!

Day Thirty

Congratulations! This is the last day of the thirty-day start-up program! I hope you've consistently followed along, learned new ideas and ways, tried them, and made them your own.

Don't stop now, by any means. Keep doing what you've been doing. Remember, this isn't a program that you stop. You've built new habits of thinking, acting, being, eating, doing, surrendering, and living. Just go on, and do what you've learned to do.

If you need help:

1. Surrender and ask God to show you the way, and trust in Him 100 percent.

2. Refer to this book often, and follow the Joy of Weight Loss program day by day, for the rest of your long, joyous life!

3. Keep gathering information about yourself: your emotions, your past, your hopes and dreams. Know that you are different every day—so keep learning.

4. Keep gathering information about life: read books, the newspaper, magazines, the Internet, going to lectures, workshops, and seminars.

5. Make sure to connect with other people. Make the effort to keep friendships alive, and make new ones.

DO THIS TODAY

Ask God for forgiveness and the power to receive it. *Know that you're supposed to be perfectly imperfect so you can keep learning by making mistakes!*

TODAY'S MENU

Today is a joy-filled day of celebration so let's rejoice in eating ordinary food in healthy moderation, having what you like!

Breakfast

M E N U	PROTEIN	GRAIN	FRUIT or VEGETABLE
A bowl of cereal	Milk (1 cup)	Cereal (1 oz. about ¾ cup average)	Banana, cut-up

- To drink, you may have coffee or tea, with a shot of milk in it, and a teaspoon of sugar if you wish.

- Don't forget—drink a big glass (eight to ten ounce) of water with your breakfast.

- Enjoy a moment of silence before you eat, appreciating all you have and realizing that feeding yourself is serious, important, and joyous. Then, eat slowly, savoring and enjoying each bite.

- Make sure to wait twenty minutes after your last bite to feel satisfied. You will feel that you've had enough.

Mid-Morning Snack

M E N U	PROTEIN	GRAIN	FRUIT or VEGETABLE
	Sardines (2 to 3 ozs.)	Cheddar crackers (5 small, approx.)	Green pepper slices (½ cup)

- DRINK: One large (eight to ten ounce) glass of water.

Lunch

MENU	PROTEIN	GRAIN	FRUIT or VEGETABLE
Veggie bake	Grated cheeses: Cheddar, Mozzarella, Parmesan on top (1½ ozs)	Bread cubes (1 slice)	Italian tomatoes, okra, snow peas, zucchini, eggplant (½ cup)— bake everything together

- **DRINK:** One large (eight to ten ounce) glass of water.

Afternoon Snack

MENU	PROTEIN	GRAIN	FRUIT or VEGETABLE
		A bowl of rice, with soy sauce (½ cup)	

- **DRINK:** One large (eight to ten ounce) glass of water.

Dinner

MENU	PROTEIN	GRAIN	FRUIT or VEGETABLE
Barbecue chicken "soul-food" dinner	Grilled chicken breast and leg: (2 ozs.) with barbeque sauce	Baked beans (1 cup). Could be either grain, vegetable or protein, here it's a carb.	Potato salad with chopped celery and pickles (¾ cup)

- **DRINK:** One large (eight to ten ounce) glass of water.

Evening Snack

MENU	PROTEIN	GRAIN	FRUIT or VEGETABLE
		Graham crackers (2 small)	Apple juice (¾ cup) in crushed ice

- **DRINK:** One large (eight to ten ounce) glass of water.

TODAY'S ACTIVITY

Thirty minutes of swimming or water dancing, water aerobics, or water jogging.

PRAYER AND MEDITATION

Thirty minutes of silence. See if you can do it! Sit in a comfortable chair or on the floor on a rug or pillow, legs crossed. Close your eyes. Use the technique that I taught you where you drift up to space and then everything disappears. Sit there, peacefully, letting all thoughts float by you one by one, not clinging to any of them. Don't try to eliminate any thoughts or feelings—that's impossible. Just don't attach to them or let them develop.

Sit in silence. Feel God's presence inside you. Feel the connection to everything that He has loved into existence. Just sit there and bask in His loving grace. There. Alive. Thriving. Well. Feel the Joy.

Now slowly return to earth, once it is time. Float back down, back to living fully, alive and well, in your life. Be new today. Thank God for your life. Amen.

The Joy of Weight Loss
Menu Ideas

When you make the effort to think good thoughts and stop depreciating yourself, you are getting better. Every time you see God in others, every time you're empathic and helpful—you are choosing joy.

When you finally realize that this life, this work, this situation, these turmoils and trials, and these unbelievable experiences of good and bad are there to help you become whole—then you begin to experience lasting joy. This is because you've found the pure, ultimate source of all joy—and that is God.

Some Food Ideas For You To Choose From

Here are some food combinations you may like. I give them to you as illustration of The Joy of Weight Loss Eating Plan. They are only ideas as to the types of meals and how much to eat at one sitting... not what you must eat. Notice that there are three columns for each meal and snack: protein, grain, fruit/vegetable.

Breakfast (choose one row or mix and match)

M E N U	PROTEIN	GRAIN	FRUIT or VEGETABLE
A bowl of cereal	Milk (I cup)	Cereal (I oz., about ¾ cup average)	Banana, cut-up
Fruit yogurt and toast	Yogurt (I cup)	Toast (I slice)	Chopped pineapple (½ cup)
Western egg/muffin sandwich	2 eggs, scrambled	English muffin	Cut-up onion, pepper, mushroom (½ cup)
Hot oatmeal	Milk (I cup)	Cooked oatmeal (½ cup)	Raisins (¼ cup)
Grilled cheese bagel	Cheese (1½oz.) natural, or processed (2 oz., about 2 slices)	Small bagel, toasted (with cheese melted)	Grilled vegetables: onions, tomato, peppers, mushrooms (½ cup)
Sausage biscuit	Sausage, meat or veggie (2 to 3 oz)	Biscuit	Orange juice (¾ cup)
Waffles and ham	Ham, meat or veggie (2 oz. slice)	Waffle	Fruit spread (½ cup, unsweetened)
European	Sliced assorted cheeses (2 slices)	Rye flat bread (I slice)	
French toast and egg	2 eggs: I for the batter dip, I fried or scrambled	I slice bread	Add a topping of fruit (chopped, ½ cup)
Belgian scrambled egg and waffles	2 eggs, scrambled	I Belgian waffle (fresh or frozen)	Chopped onion, green pepper and carrots (add to the scrambled egg).

Morning Snack (choose one row, or mix and match)

M E N U	PROTEIN	GRAIN	FRUIT or VEGETABLE
	(at only I snack time per day)		
	Peanuts (⅓ cup or 2 tbs)	Popcorn (I cup, approx., not buttered)	Apple juice (¾ cup)
	Cheese (2 ozs. processed, 1½ natural)	Crackers (5 approximately)	Carrot sticks (½ cup)

M E N U	PROTEIN	GRAIN	FRUIT or VEGETABLE
	Toasted soybeans ($^1\!/_3$ cup)	Pretzels (7 small, 2 big)	Cherry tomatoes ($^1\!/_2$ cup)
	Cottage cheese (1$^1\!/_2$ ozs.)	Bread (1 slice)	Vegetable juice ($^3\!/_4$ cup)
	Turkey (2 to 3 ozs.)	Baked corn chips (10)	Apple (medium)
	Milk (1 cup)	Cereal (1 oz. $^3\!/_4$ cup avg.)	Pear slices ($^1\!/_2$ cup)
	Leftover lamb kabob (2 to 3 ozs.)	Leftover rice ($^1\!/_2$ cup)	Grapes ($^1\!/_2$ cup)
	Bouillon (1 cup)	Roll	Applesauce ($^1\!/_2$ cup)
	Chick and kidney beans in the salad ($^1\!/_2$ cup)	Flat bread (2 sticks)	Three-bean salad (1 cup = $^1\!/_2$ cup vegetables, $^1\!/_2$ cup beans)
	Yogurt dip with herbs (1 cup)	pumpernickel bread (1 slice)	Crudités: slices of red, yellow and green peppers, carrots, etc. ($^1\!/_2$ cup approx.)

Lunch (choose one row, or mix and match)

M E N U	PROTEIN	GRAIN	FRUIT or VEGETABLE
Sandwich: grilled	Grilled chicken (2 ozs.)	Small bun	Lettuce and tomato, pickles on the side
Sandwich: tuna salad	Tuna salad (2 ozs.)	Small roll	Lettuce and tomato, pickles and carrot sticks on the side
Sandwich: peanut butter and jelly	Peanut butter (2 tbs)	Bread (1 slice) —or skip the grain part of your next snack and have 2	Fruit spread, unsweetened, preferably ($^1\!/_4$ cup)
Salad: nicoise	Anchovies or tuna fish (2 ozs.)	Croutons (1 oz or $^1\!/_2$ cup)	Raw spinach and lettuce ($^1\!/_2$ cup), potatoes, tomatoes ($^1\!/_4$ cup)
Salad: fruit and cottage cheese	Cottage cheese (1$^1\!/_2$ ozs.)	Whole wheat bread (1 slice)	Fresh peach, orange, apple, pear, banana slices (1 medium, or $^1\!/_2$ cup chopped)

MENU	PROTEIN	GRAIN	FRUIT or VEGETABLE
Salad: tossed	Shredded cheese (1 1/2 ozs.)	Croutons (1 oz or ½ cup)	Raw spinach and lettuce (½ cup), tomatoes, celery (¼ cup)
Pizza with veggies	Shredded cheese (1½ ozs.)	Crust (1 slice)	Tomato sauce. Onions, green pepper, broccoli, tomatoes (½ cup)
Hamburger or veggie burger	Patty—beef, turkey, or veggie (2 ozs.)	Small bun	Lettuce and tomato, pickles on the side
Soup: chicken vegetable	Chicken: cut-up (2 ozs.)	Pasta or barley, (½ cup)	Vegetables, cooked cut-up (½ cup)
Salad bar	Beans: chick, kidney, canoli, black-eyed (1 cup)	Croutons (½ cup)	leafy greens (¾ cup), add chopped, mixed veggies: carrot, beets, radishes, cucumber, tomato, zucchini, etc. (¼ cup)
Spanish roast chicken	Roasted chicken, spicy herb marinade (2 to 3 ozs.)	Yellow Rice (½ cup)	Mixed Vegetables, cooked (½ cup): plantain, green olive, tomato, hot peppers.
Pasta florentine	Diced mozzarella (2 ozs.)	Pasta shells, cooked (½ cup)	Cooked spinach and garlic (in the pasta)
Wrap: turkey breast	Turkey Breast (⅔ ozs. sliced)	Flour tortilla (1)	Shredded lettuce, sliced tomato and dill pickles (½ cup)
Turkey chili	Turkey cubes, kidney beans (2 to 3 ozs.)	Cornbread (2 x 2-inch square)	Cooked corn, tomatillos, tomatoes, black olives (½ cup)
Veggie bake	Grated cheeses: cheddar, mozzarella, parmesan on top (1½ ozs)	Bread cubes (1 slice)	Italian tomatoes, okra, snow peas, zucchini, eggplant (½ cup)—bake everything together
Fast food burger and fries (rare treat!)	1 burger (¼ lb., or 2 to 3 ozs.)	Bun	French fries (10), and ketchup

Afternoon / Evening Snack *(choose one row, or mix and match)*

M E N U	PROTEIN	GRAIN	FRUIT or VEGETABLE
	(at only 1 snack time per day)		
	Brie cheese (1½ oz. natural)	Oat-bran crackers (5, average)	Kiwi fruit (medium)
	Cashew nuts (2 tbs)	Belgian wafers (5 small, average)	Peach (medium)
	Tuna (2 to 3 ozs.)	Slice pumpernickel bread	Cucumber (½ cup)
	Yogurt (1 cup)	Vanilla wafers (5 small, approx.)	Banana (medium)
	Peanut butter (2 tbs)	Saltines (6, approximately)	Celery (2 stalks, or ½ cup approx.)
	Muenster cheese (1½ oz.)	Melba toast (2 small slices)	Tangerine (medium)
	Pea or bean dip (chick peas, black or kidney beans mashed —½ cup, in ½ cup yogurt)	Baked tortilla chips (6 chips)	Mixed into dip: shredded carrots, cucumbers, radishes, Tabasco or jalapeno sauce (½ cup total)
	Pork filling in the Dim Sum (2 to 3 ozs.)	Dim sum—dumpling dough (3 approx.)	Lychees (½ cup)
	2 hard-boiled eggs	Rice cakes (2)	Dried apricots (¼ cup)
		Pretzel nuggets (10)	apple-cranberry juice (¾ cup)
	A cup of milk	Dinner roll (1)	Peach slices (½ cup)
	A cup of milk	Bowl of ready-to-eat cereal (¾ cup)	Raisins, dried fruit (¼ cup)

Dinner

MENU	PROTEIN	GRAIN	FRUIT or VEGETABLE
Lasagna	Ground beef or TVP* and shredded cheese (2 ozs.)	Pasta: cooked lasagna noodles ($^1/_2$ cup)	Tomato sauce ($^3/_4$ cup)
Spaghetti and meatballs	Ground beef or tofu (2 ozs.)	Pasta: cooked noodles ($^1/_2$ cup)	Applesauce ($^1/_2$ cup) (for dessert)
Southern fish supper	Broiled catfish (2 ozs.)	Cornbread (1 slice)	Collard greens ($^1/_2$ cup), cooked
burrito	Ground beef, turkey, or soy protein (2 ozs.)	Soft flour or corn tortilla	Shredded tomato, lettuce, onions, olives, hot or sweet peppers ($^1/_2$ cup)
Chinese chicken chow mien	Shredded chicken (2 ozs.), in sauce	Chow mien noodles ($^1/_2$ cup)	Bok choy (Chinese cabbage) water chestnuts, broccoli ($^1/_2$ cup)
Thai shrimp and vegetables	Cooked shrimp and chopped peanut (2 ozs.), in sauce	Thai "glass" noodles ($^1/_2$ cup)	Scallions, snow peas, shredded carrot ($^1/_2$ cup)
Grilled cheese sandwich	Cheddar or American cheese (2 slices)	Whole wheat or rye bread (1 slice or skip the grain part of your next snack and have 2)	Strawberries ($^1/_2$ cup)
Pasta primavera	Grated parmesan cheese (1 oz.) white canoli beans ($^1/_4$ cup)	Pasta—try angel hair—($^1/_2$ cup), cooked	Chopped vegetables: carrots, broccoli, spinach, onions, green beans, squash ($^1/_2$ cup)
Barbecue chicken "soul-food" dinner	Grilled chicken breast and leg (2 ozs.) with barbeque sauce	Baked beans (1 cup (could be either grain, or protein, here it's a carb.)	Potato salad with chopped celery and pickles ($^1/_2$ cup)
Turkey and trimmings	Sliced roasted turkey (2 to 3 ozs.)	Stuffing (1, 2-inch square)	Baked potato (1 medium or $^1/_2$ cup mashed)
Chicken pot pie	Sliced chicken (2 to 3 ozs.)	Crust (about the equivalent of a slice of bread)	Mixed vegetables in vegetable bouillon ($^1/_2$ cup cooked)
Jewish kosher	Shwarma, ground beef or lamb (2 to 3 ozs.)	Matzos (unleavened bread, like crackers)	Shredded, pickled radish and beets ($^1/_2$ cup)

* TVP = Texturized Vegetable Protein

Tortellini with peas	Cheese tortellini (½ cup)	1 dinner roll	Cooked peas (mixed in, in vegetable bouillon ½ cup)
Roast Long Island duckling	Duckling (2 to 3 ounces)	Carrot muffin	Chopped cherry and apple medley, in unsweetened juice (½ cup)
Indian bean masala	Curried chick peas and kidney beans (1 cup)	Brown rice (½ cup)	Cooked green peas, tomato, onion, garlic (½ cup)
Polish feast	Pierogies—potato and cheese,(¾ cup approx.)	Challa—egg—bread (1 slice)	Sauerkraut (½ cup)
Stuffed sole	Sole fish fillets, baked (2 to 3 ozs.)	Bread crumbs (¼ cup) and marsala wine (1 tablespoon)	Fresh spinach stuffing with onion, mushroom, garlic, oregano (½ cup)

The Joy of Weight Loss
Daily Checklist

(MAKE COPIES AND USE EVERY DAY)

I allowed Myself Joy ❐

Surrender / Reflection / Meditation ❐

USDA Food Pyramid, Food Group Servings

Grains ❐ ❐ ❐ ❐ ❐ ❐

Vegetables ❐ ❐ ❐

Fruits ❐ ❐

Proteins: Meat/Fish/Beans/Nuts ❐ ❐

Proteins: Dairy Group ❐ ❐

Silence Before Eating ❐ ❐ ❐ ❐ ❐ ❐

Pleasurable Activity _____

How Many Minutes of Activity?

10 ❐   20 ❐   30 ❐   40 ❐   50 ❐   60 ❐

I Helped Someone ❐

I Shared My Feelings and Experiences ❐

I Listened to Others ❐

I Took Time to Learn Something New ❐

I Felt the Presence of God ❐   I Saw God in Others ❐

Citations are organized by page number:

18: An old saying. Quoted in Evan Esar, ed. *20,000 Quips and Quotes.* Doubleday: Garden City, NY. (1968).

19: Abraham Lincoln. Quoted in Evan Esar, ed. *20,000 Quips and Quotes.* Doubleday: Garden City, NY. (1968).

20: Karen Horney. Quoted in Rosalie Maggio, ed. *Quotations by Women.* Beacon Press: Boston (1994).

21: Djuna Barnes. Rosalie Maggio, ed. *Quotations by Women.* Beacon Press: Boston (1994).

22: Khalil Gibran. Quoted in Quotation Archive (Internet).

23: Colette. Rosalie Maggio, ed. *Quotations by Women.* Beacon Press: Boston (1994).

23: Sara Teasdale. Rosalie Maggio, ed. *Quotations by Women.* Beacon Press: Boston (1994).

23: Psalm 36. *Holy Bible: King James Version.*

24: Ralph Waldo Emerson. Quoted in W.H. Auden and Louis Kronenberger, eds. *The Viking Book of Aphorisms,* Viking: New York (1993).

25: Ramana Maharshi: Quoted in Stephen Mitchell. *The Gospel According to Jesus: A New Translation and Guide to His Essential Teachings for Believers and Unbelievers.* HarperCollins: New York (1993).

26: Mahatma Gandhi: Quoted in Stephen Mitchell. *The Gospel According to Jesus: A New Translation and Guide to His Essential Teachings for Believers and Unbelievers.* HarperCollins: New York (1993).

26: "I remember one day..." by Leo Tolstoy. Quoted in William James. *The Varieties of Religious Experience.* Simon and Schuster: New York (1997).

27: His Holiness, the Dalai Lama. His Holiness the Dalai Lama and Howard C. Cutler, MD. *The Art of Happiness: A Handbook for Living.* Riverhead: New York (1998).

27: "A few weeks after..." by Jacques Lusseyran. Quoted in Stephen Mitchell. *The Gospel According to Jesus: A New Translation and Guide to His Essential Teachings for Believers and Unbelievers.* HarperCollins: New York (1993).

27: Exodus 3:13–14. The Torah: *The Five Books of Moses*. Philadelphia: Jewish Publication Society (1992).

29: "I was walking again..." by David Brainerd. Quoted in William James. *The Varieties of Religious Experience*. Simon and Schuster: New York (1997).

30: "I have had many nice moments..." by Muhammad Ali. Quoted on *Muslim.net*. www.muslim.net/islam/mohamed.htm.

31: Carl Jung. C. J. Jung. *Memories, Dreams, Reflections*. Vintage: New York (1961).

32: "I longed to..." by St. Augustine. Augustine. *Confessions*. Translated with an introduction by R.S. Pine-Coffin. Penguin: New York (1961).

34: Angelus Silesius. Quoted in Stephen Mitchell, ed. *The Enlightened Heart: An Anthology of Sacred Poetry*. Harper and Row: New York (1989).

34: Søren Kierkegaard. Quoted in Evan Esar, ed. *20,000 Quips and Quotes*. Doubleday: Garden City, NY. (1968).

35: Psalm 23: *Holy Bible: King James Version*.

36: St. Augustine on Psalm 37. Quoted in Diocese of Peoria, IL. "Evangelization, Spiritual Catechesis and Ongoing Conversion: The Basic Elements of an Adult Spiritual Life." (Internet)

36: Psalm 16: *Holy Bible: King James Version*.

37: The Holy Qu'ran: *Holy Qu'ran*. King Fahd Holy Cur-an Printing Complex: Mushaf Al-Madinah An-Nabawiyah.

38: Zohar. Quoted in Roy Frank, ed. *Webster's Quotationary*. Random House: New York (1998).

38: "In the National Weight Control...." Mary Klem, *et al.* "A Descriptive Study of Individuals Successful at Long-Term Maintenance of Substantial Weight Loss." **American Journal of Clinical Nutrition** (1997) 66:239–46.

38: George Bernard Shaw. Quotation Archive (Internet).

39: "Obesity treatment programs...." Martha L. Skender, Ken Goodrick, *et al.*, "Comparison of 2-year weight loss trends in behavioral treatments of obesity: diet, exercise, and combination interventions" **Journal of the American Dietetic Association**. (April 1996) 96:4.

40: Virginia Woolf. Quotation Archive (Internet).

46: Hippocrates Magazine. Quoted in Roy Frank, ed. *Webster's Quotationary*. Random House: New York (1998)

47: "It's not the minutes...." Quoted in Evan Esar, ed. *20,000 Quips and Quotes*. Doubleday: Garden City, NY. (1968).

48: Frederick Buechner. Quoted in Roy Frank, ed. *Webster's Quotationary*. Random House: New York (1998)

49: Grain Group Serving Sizes: USDA. "The 2000 Dietary Guidelines for Americans, 5th edition." United States Department of Agriculture and U.S. Department of Health and Human Services.

50: Vegetable Group Serving Sizes. USDA. "The 2000 Dietary Guidelines for Americans, 5th edition." United States Department of Agriculture and U.S. Department of Health and Human Services.

51: Fruit Group Serving Sizes. USDA. "The 2000 Dietary Guidelines for Americans, 5th edition." United States Department of Agriculture and U.S. Department of Health and Human Services.

52: Bertrand Russell. Quoted in Evan Esar, ed. *20,000 Quips and Quotes*. Doubleday: Garden City, NY. (1968).

53: Meat and Beans Group Serving Sizes. USDA. "The 2000 Dietary Guidelines for Americans, 5th edition." United States Department of Agriculture and U.S. Department of Health and Human Services.

55: Milk Group Serving Sizes. USDA. "The 2000 Dietary Guidelines for Americans, 5th edition." United States Department of Agriculture and U.S. Department of Health and Human Services.

56: "Young children with lactase deficiency...." National Institutes of Health. Publication No. 98-2751 (April 1994). Updated: November 1998.

56: Saying (Vermont). Quoted in Roy Frank, ed. *Webster's Quotationary*. Random House: New York (1998).

65: National Academy of Sciences. National Academy of Sciences. "Summary: Weighing the Options—Criteria for Evaluating Weight Management Programs." **Journal of the American Dietetic Association** (1995) 95:96–105.

66: University of California Wellness Center. Timothy P. White and editors of the University of California Wellness Letter. *The Wellness Guide to Lifelong Fitness*. Rebus: New York (1993).

67: Edward Stanley. Quoted in Evan Esar, ed. *20,000 Quips and Quotes*. Doubleday: Garden City, NY. (1968).

70: "Ten minutes of exercise...." Zelasco, Chester J., Ph.D., "Exercise for Weight Loss: What are the Facts?" **Journal of the American Dietetic Association**, December (1995) 95: 1416.

70: "Observe your dog...." Quoted in Evan Esar, ed. *20,000 Quips and Quotes*. Doubleday: Garden City, NY. (1968).

71: Thomas Jefferson. Quoted in Roy Frank, ed. *Webster's Quotationary*. Random House: New York (1998).

71: "On the National Weight Control...." Mary Klem, *et al.* "A Descriptive Study of Individuals Successful at Long-Term Maintenance of Substantial Weight Loss." **American Journal of Clinical Nutrition** (1997) 66:239–46.

73: Henry David Thoreau. Quoted in Roy Frank, ed. *Webster's Quotationary*. Random House: New York (1998).

73: Sarah Leah Grafstein. Quoted in Rosalie Maggio, ed. *Quotations by Women*. Beacon Press: Boston (1994).

74: Ralph Waldo Emerson. Quoted in Roy Frank, ed. *Webster's Quotationary*. Random House: New York (1998).

76: Benedict Spinoza. Quoted in Dorothy Berkley Phillips, Elizabeth Boyden Howes, Lucille M. Nixon, eds. *The Choice Is Always Ours: The Classic Anthology On The Spiritual Way*. HarperCollins: New York (1989).

77: Herbert Benson, MD. Herbert Benson, MD. *Timeless Healing: The Power and Biology of Belief*. Scribner: New York (1996).

77: Carl Jung. C. G. Jung. *Modern Man in Search of a Soul*. Translated by W.S. Dell and Cary F. Baynes. Harvest Books: New York (1933).

78: Meister Johannes Eckhart. Quoted in Dorothy Berkley Phillips, Elizabeth Boyden Howes, Lucille M. Nixon, eds. *The Choice Is Always Ours: The Classic Anthology On The Spiritual Way*. HarperCollins: New York (1989).

79: Ramban. Reproduced from "Ramban: 'A Letter For The Ages'" by Rabbi Avrohom Chaim Feurer with permission from the copyright holders Artscroll/Mesorah Publications Ltd, Brooklyn, NY.

80: Tung-Shan. Quoted in Stephen Mitchell, ed. *The Enlightened Heart: An Anthology of Sacred Poetry*. Harper and Row: New York (1989)

80: Erica Jong. Quoted in Rosalie Maggio, ed. *Quotations by Women*. Beacon Press: Boston (1994).

82: Channing Pollack. Quoted in Quotation Archive (Internet).

83: His Holiness, the Dalai Lama. Quoted in Quotation Archive (Internet).

82: Cynthia Heimel. Quoted in Rosalie Maggio, ed. *Quotations by Women*. Beacon Press: Boston (1994).

85: Ntozake Shange. Quoted in Rosalie Maggio, ed. *Quotations by Women*. Beacon Press: Boston (1994).

87: Carl Jung. C. G. Jung. *The Portable Jung*. Edited by Joseph Campbell. Viking: New York (1971).

89: Matthew 6. *Holy Bible: King James Version*. Abradale Press: New York (1965)

94: Johann Wolfgang von Goethe. Quoted in Roy Frank, ed. *Webster's Quotationary*. Random House: New York (1998).

96: Ralph Waldo Emerson. Quoted in Roy Frank, ed. *Webster's Quotationary*. Random House: New York (1998).

97: Johann Wolfgang von Goethe. Quoted in Dorothy Berkley Phillips, Elizabeth Boyden Howes, Lucille M. Nixon, eds. *The Choice Is Always Ours: The Classic Anthology On The Spiritual Way*. HarperCollins: New York (1989).

99: Anonymous. Quoted in Herbert Benson, MD. *Timeless Healing: The Power and Biology of Belief*. Scribner: New York (1996).